Pocket Guide to
MEDICATIONS
USED IN
DERMATOLOGY

Second Edition

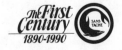

The First Century
1890-1990
SANS TACHE

Pocket Guide to
MEDICATIONS
USED IN
DERMATOLOGY

Second Edition

Andrew J. Scheman, M.D.

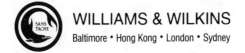

WILLIAMS & WILKINS
Baltimore • Hong Kong • London • Sydney

Editor: G. Terry Minton
Associate Editor: M. Fran Witthauer
Copy Editor: Janis Oppelt
Designer: Dan Pfisterer
Production Coordinator: Charles E. Zeller

Accurate indications, adverse reactions, and dosage schedules for drugs are provided in this book, but it is possible that they may change. The reader is urged to review the package information data of the manufacturers of the medications mentioned.

Printed in the United States of America

Library of Congress Cataloging-in-Publication Data

Scheman, Andrew J.
    Pocket guide to medications used in dermatology / by Andrew J. Scheman.—2nd ed.
        mp. cm.
        ISBN 0–683–07591–8
    1. Dermatologic agents–Handbooks, manuals, etc. 2. Skin—Diseases—Chemotherapy—Handbooks, manuals, etc. I. Title.
    [DNLM: 1. Dermatologic Agents—therapeutic use—handbooks.
2. Skin Diseases—drug therapy—handbooks. WR 39 S323p]
RL801.S44   1989
615.778—dc20
DNLM/DLC
for Library of Congress

                                            89–16661
                                                 CIP

Page

Page

Keep this book handy: you will use it often! Dr. Andrew Scheman has catalogued a vast array of topical and systemic dermatologic medications and listed not only the brand names but also the generic names, concentrations, vehicles, sizes, and dosages. When used in conjunction with knowledge of drug mechanisms, indications, contraindications, side effects, and dose variabilities, this information should greatly aid us all in treating patients with various skin diseases.

When I began treating patients with dermatologic disorders, I was confounded by the vast array of formulations and preparations available to me. One teacher told me I would only need to learn a few and that these few would be adequate weapons to treat all skin diseases. He was both right and wrong. A few may be adequate, but many are better. Though many formulations are similar, they frequently are not quite identical. There are subtle and nonsubtle reasons that one might choose one preparation over another. Accordingly, I use a large array of proprietary preparations and occasionally compound preparations as well. I think it was because I confounded Dr. Scheman during his dermatologic training that he began to tabulate and list various topical agents and their subtle differences. From that grew this book. I am honored that he asked me to write this foreword for the second edition.

I think you will find here a very useful, concise reference. Appropriate medications can be selected for appropriate indications while a patient is in the office. A review at home of the preparations available and their similarities and differences helps hone prescribing skills.

In summary, this book provides specific data on therapy. If anyone thinks dermatologic therapy is simple, this book testifies to the contrary. With this book, if we don't know, we can look it up. Dr. Scheman has provided us with a real tool for formulating effective treatment regimens.

Mark V. Dahl, M.D.
Professor of Dermatology
University of Minnesota Medical School

I keep two booklets in my white coat, and this is one of them. There is no other single source of dermatologic product information that is as comprehensive, convenient, and practical. This second edition incorporates numerous and valuable features that go beyond mere product listing by including such details as the active ingredients of sunscreens, the base ingredients of moisturizers, and side effects and suggested laboratory monitoring of a number of potent internal medications. Dr. Scheman has provided an immensely valuable resource for the dermatologist, and I thank him for this booklet almost daily. (The second book I carry is *A Guide to Drug Eruptions* by W. Bruinsma, The File of Medicines, Netherlands).

Stanford I. Lamberg, M.D.
Associate Professor of Dermatology
Johns Hopkins University

Of all medications that a physician is likely to encounter, a thorough understanding of dermatologic products is perhaps most elusive. There are several reasons for this problem. First, there is no single source that lists all of these products. The most widely used reference, the *Physician's Desk Reference*, is useful but notably lacks many dermatologic products. In addition, there are numerous nonprescription dermatologic products, and many of these are not listed in the standard reference books. Finally, medical schools spend little or no time on dermatologic therapy and, therefore, most physicians learn this information primarily from observing other physicians. The end result is that most nondermatologists and many dermatologists are only aware of a small proportion of the tools available for treating skin problems.

The response to the first edition of *Pocket Guide to Medications Used in Dermatology* has been outstanding. This second edition retains the format of the earlier edition but has been improved in several ways. The new edition remains a comprehensive pocket-sized handbook to dermatologic products and their usage. The charts are designed for quick reference and easy comparison of available choices.

New features include an extremely useful section on bases and vehicles containing essential principles needed to properly choose topical corticosteroids, emollients, and other topical products to achieve optimal response. The individual charts on corticosteroids and emollients have been expanded to include information on bases and potential sensitizing ingredients. A simplified six-class model of topical corticosteroid strength has been used to assess relative strength of these products. The emollient section also has information on potential comedogenic ingredients and the results of rabbit ear assays of overall product comedogenicity. Since many patients use emollient products obtained from companies marketing through department stores, representative products from these companies have been added.

New charts have been added on topical antihistamines, antiseborrheics, intralesional or intramuscular corticosteroids, debriding agents, fish oils, ophthalmics, otic preparations, and miscellaneous medications. Detailed prescribing information has been added on cyclosporine, dapsone, etretinate, griseofulvin, hydroxychloroquine, isotretinoin, ketoconazole, methotrexate, and methoxsalen. Also the relative strength of tar products has been better standardized in this edition.

All prescription products are now marked "Rx" for easy identification. Also, the index has been improved by italicizing generic preparations in order to separate them from brand-name products. These improvements should make this second edition even more useful than the preceding edition.

I gratefully acknowledge the extensive expert data processing and technical work done by my research assistant, David Severson. The support and encouragement provided by Dr. Stanford I. Lamberg throughout this project is also greatly appreciated. I wish to thank Dr. Joel Sequeira of Schering Corporation for his collaboration on the pharmacology of topical bases and vehicles. The assistance of Dr. Robin Winter-Sperry, Stephen Trynowski, and Dan Carlson of Schering Corporation was also appreciated.

I welcome any constructive comments and suggestions and would like to encourage drug company representatives to provide information on products being added to or deleted from the market, formulation changes, and products inadvertently omitted from the current edition.

Correspondence may be directed to:

> Andrew Scheman, M.D.
> 1400 Golf Road, Suite 126
> Des Plaines, Illinois 60016

At every pharmacy, the cost to the patient is calculated using a formula, and, usually, a pharmacy charge is added to the result. For example, at the University of Minnesota (9/85):

$$\text{Patient cost} = (\text{pharmacy cost} \times 1.3) + \$3.70$$

One large prescription is much less expensive than the same amount of medicine given using refills, since the pharmacy charge is added to each refill. This is particularly true of inexpensive medicines where the pharmacy charge can represent most of the patient cost. For example:

	Inexpensive Medicine		
	Drug A	Drug A	Drug A
	#30	#90	#30 2RF
Pharm cost per tablet	$.0093	.0093	.0093
No. of tablets	× 30	× 90	× 90
Total pharm cost	$ .28	.84	.84
Pharm charge	$3.70	3.70	11.10
Patient cost	$3.98	4.54	11.94

Cost Effectiveness for Chronic Patients

(1) Note how the price of 30 tablets of Drug A is not much different from the cost of 90 tablets, since the majority of the patient cost is pharmacy charges. This is not true of Drug B. *Order in larger quantities whenever possible.*

(2) Note how the price of 90 tablets of Drug A more than doubles when ordered as 30 pills with two refills. The difference noted with Drug B is also significant but not quite as large. *Avoid refills as much as possible.*

(3) Note that Drug A and Drug B are fairly similar in price in small quantities but that prices diverge when the drugs are ordered in larger quantities. *In small quantity, the price difference between drugs is minimized.*

(4) There may also be a bulk discount for certain topical drugs. For example:

> 0.1% triamcinolone cream 15 grams: $ 0.04/gram
> 0.1% triamcinolone cream 240 grams: $0.0246/gram
> (UMN, 9/85)

Expensive Medicine		
Drug B	Drug B	Drug B
#30	#90	#30 2RF
$.0619	.0619	.0619
× 30	× 90	× 90
$1.86	5.57	5.57
3.70	3.70	11.10
$5.56	9.27	16.67

Many patients undergoing acne therapy are on oral contraceptives. Some oral contraceptives improve acne substantially while others aggravate it. Generally, pills with higher estrogen content have the most positive effect on acne, however, this must be carefully weighed against the potential for increased side effects associated with these medications. In addition, products with nonandrogenic progestogens (such as ethynodiol diacetate or norethynodrel) are preferred for patients with acne. With the recent elimination of Ovulen and Enovid-E from the market, there are only a few choices remaining that contain nonandrogenic progestogens. Products with more androgenic progestogens (such as norgestrel) should be avoided by acne patients. Many feel that a dose of 100 mcg of ethinyl estradiol daily is required to suppress severe acne. At this dosage, 50 to 70% of women with recalcitrant cystic acne will improve in 3 to 4 months. Mestranol is approximately two thirds the potency of ethinyl estradiol.

Oral Contraceptives with Nonandrogenic Progestogens:

Brand Name	Estrogen	Progestin	Preparation
Rx Demulen 1/35	35 mcg ethinyl estradiol	1 mg ethynodiol diacetate	Pkgs of 21 or 28
Rx Demulen 1/50	50 mcg ethinyl estradiol	1 mg ethynodiol diacetate	Pkgs of 21 or 28
Rx Enovid 5 mg	75 mcg mestranol	5 mg norethynodrel	Bottle of 100
Rx Enovid 10 mg	150 mcg mestranol	9.85 mg norethynodrel	Bottle of 50
Rx Estinyl	50 mcg ethinyl estradiol	—	Bottles of 100 or 250

(1) *21 pill schedule:* Take 1 pill every day for 3 weeks (starting the first package on the Sunday after menstrual period begins). Skip 1 week. Repeat each month.

(2) *28 pill schedule:* Take 1 pill every day (starting the first package on the Sunday after menstrual period starts).

ISOTRETINOIN (13-cis retinoic acid) (Accutane)

DOSAGE (Acne):

1. Start with 0.5 to 1.0 mg/kg/d.
2. Dosages as low as 0.1 mg/kg/d will clear most patients but recurrence requiring retreatment is increased with lower dosages.
   a. 0.1 mg/kg/d–42% required retreatment
   b. 0.5 mg/kg/d–20% required retreatment
   c. 1.0 mg/kg/d–10% required retreatment
3. May need up to 2 mg/kg/d for severe truncal involvement.
4. Treat up to 20 weeks but can stop treatment earlier if cyst count is 70% reduced from baseline.
5. A second course can be initiated, if needed, after an 8-week period off therapy.

LAB TESTS:

1. Pregnancy test:
   a. Need negative test within 2 weeks of initiation of treatment and then at least monthly during treatment.
   b. Need two forms of birth control during treatment and until 1 month after treatment.
   c. Begin Accutane on second or third day of menstrual period.

2. Triglycerides (fasting, 36 hours after last alcohol ingestion), liver function tests:
   a. Obtain at baseline and weeks 2 and 4 or 3 and 6.
   b. Can then stop monitoring if values are normal.
   c. Often obtained at end of treatment also.
   d. Most likely elevated in patients with personal or family history of diabetes mellitus, obesity, or heavy alcohol consumption.

3. Other tests: Some physicians also monitor complete blood count, urinalysis, glucose, and cholesterol.

CONTRAINDICATIONS:

1. Pregnancy, nursing mothers.
2. Paraben allergy (capsules contain parabens).

INTERACTIONS:

1. Tetracycline increases incidence of pseudotumor cerebri.
2. Vitamin A increases incidence of toxicity in general.

HOW SUPPLIED:

10, 20, 40 mg capsules

ISOTRETINOIN (13-cis retinoic acid) (Accutane) (continued)

SIDE EFFECTS: (*Denotes side effects that require stopping treatment)

Organ System	Side Effect
Cutaneous and related symptoms	Chelitis Dry skin, nose, mouth, eyes Rash Hair thinning Skin infection Photosensitivity Palmoplantar desquamation *Exuberant granulation tissue formation Pyogenic granuloma
Ocular	Conjunctivitis Poor night vision *Corneal opacities Irritation from contact lenses
Musculoskeletal and Neurologic	Bone and joint pain Headache Diffuse idiopathic skeletal hyperostosis (DISH) Premature epiphysis closure CNS symptoms (various) *Pseudotumor cerebri
Gastrointestinal	Nausea, vomiting *Inflammatory bowel disease
Other	*Birth defects
Laboratory	Elevated sedimentation rate Elevated triglycerides (mild) *Elevated triglycerides (severe) Decreased high density lipoproteins *Elevated liver function tests Decreased blood count parameters White blood cells in urine Increased platelets Protein or blood in urine Elevated glucose Elevated cholesterol Elevated CPK with vigorous exercise

Occurrence	Comments
> 90%	Dose related.
< 80%	Rarely may persist; may also have skin fragility, pruritis, epistaxis.
< 10%	
< 10%	Rarely may persist.
5%	*Staph aureus* common.
5%	
5%	
—	Occurs at sites of acne lesions.
—	
40%	
—	Rarely may persist.
—	Dose related, reversible.
—	May persist.
16%	Mild to moderate; rarely may persist.
5%	
—	Dose related (mild at acne dosage), get x-rays if symptomatic
—	Dose related (infrequent at acne dosage).
—	Reported but may not be related to isotretinoin.
—	Often with concomitant tetracycline use.
5%	May present with headache, nausea, vomiting, or visual symptoms.
—	May present with abdominal pain, severe diarrhea, or rectal bleeding.
—	Affects organogenesis and causes birth defects; also may cause spontaneous abortion.
40%	Contraindicated in pregnant women.
25%	Dose related. Reversible. If 300–500, a low-fat diet, weight loss, no alcohol, lower dosage may help.
< 4%	If > 500, stopping medication often indicated if not normalized.
16%	Reversible.
15%	Mild to moderate; may be dose related; stop medication if persists and evaluate.
10–20%	
10–20%	
10–20%	
< 10%	
< 10%	
7%	Reversible. Elevations usually mild.
—	Significance unknown.

(See also: Acne Medications, Oral)
(used qd or bid unless otherwise noted)

BPO = benzoyl peroxide   HC = hydrocortisone

Brand Name	Preparation	Sizes
BENZOYL PEROXIDE:		
Acne-Aid	10% cream	54 gm
Benoxyl	5,10% lotion	30,60 ml
Rx Benzac (alcohol)*	5,10% gel	60 gm
Rx Benzac-W (water)*	2.5,5,10% gel	60 gm
Rx Benzagel (alcohol)*	5,10% gel	45,90 gm
Buf-Oxal 10	10% gel	60 gm
Clear by Design	2.5% gel	45 gm
Clearasil BP	10% lotion	30 ml
Clearasil SS Cover	10% cream	20,30 gm
Cuticura Acne	5% cream	30 gm
Rx Desquam-E (water)*	2.5,5,10% gel	45 gm
(emollient base)		
Rx Desquam-X (water)*	2.5% gel	45 gm
	5,10% gel	45,90 gm
Dry and Clear	5% lotion	30,60 ml
Dry and Clear DS	10% cream	30 gm
Fostex BPO	5,10% gel,	45 gm
	10% cream	
Loroxide	5.5% lotion	25 ml
Neutrogena Acne Mask	5% mask	60 gm
(use 20 min qd)		
Noxema Acne 12	10% lotion	30 ml
Noxzema On the Spot	10% cream	7.5 gm
(light, medium shades)		
Oxy, 5,10	5,10% lotion	30 ml
Oxy 10 Cover	10% cream cover-up	30 gm
Rx PanOxyl (alcohol)*	5,10% gel	60,120 gm
Rx PanOxyl-AQ (water)*	2.5,5,10% gel	60,120 gm
Rx Peroxin A (water)*	2.5,5,10% gel	45 gm
Rx Persa-Gel (acetone)*	5,10% gel	45,90 gm
Rx Persa-Gel W (water)*	5,10% gel	45,90 gm
pHisoAc BP	10% cream	30 gm
Propa pH	5% pads	45/box
	10% stick	1.5 gm
Stridex BP	10% lotion	30 ml
Rx Sulfoxyl (regular)	5%+2% sulfur lotion	60 ml
Rx Sulfoxyl (strong)	10%+2% sulfur lotion	60 ml
Vanoxide	5% lotion	25,50 ml
Rx Vanoxide HC	5% Lotion (+0.5%HC)	25 ml
Xerac BP5 (water)*	5% gel	45,90 gm
Xerac BP10 (water)*	10% gel	45 gm
Xerac BP	10% solution	90 ml

*BPO gels may use water, alcohol, or acetone as a solvent.

(See also: Acne Medications, Oral)
(used qd or bid unless otherwise noted)

Brand Name	Generic	Preparation	Sizes
ANTIBIOTICS:			
Rx Akne-Mycin	Erythromycin	2% ointment	25 gm
		2% solution	60 ml
Rx A/T/S	Erythromycin	2% solution	60 ml
Rx Benzamycin	Erythromycin/ BPO	3% erythromycin +5% BPO gel	23.3 gm (mix)
Rx Cleocin T	Clindamycin	1% solution	30,60,480 ml
		1% gel	7.5,30 gm
		1% lotion	60 ml
Rx Erycette	Erythromycin	2% swabs	60/box
Rx Eryderm	Erythromycin	2% solution	60 ml
Rx Erygel	Erythromycin	2% gel	30,65 gm
Rx Erymax	Erythromycin	2% solution	60,120 ml
Rx Ery-Sol	Erythromycin	2% solution	60 ml
Rx Meclan	Meclocycline	1% cream	20,45 gm
Rx Metrogel	Metronidazole	0.75% gel	30 gm
Rx Staticin	Erythromycin	1.5% solution	60 ml
Rx T-Stat	Erythromycin	2% solution	60 ml
		2% pads	60/box
Rx Topicycline	Tetracycline	solution	70 ml (mix)
KERATOLYTICS:			
Saligel	Salicyclic Acid	5% gel	60 gm
RETINOIDS:			
Rx Retin-A (use qhs)	Tretinoin	0.05% solution	28 ml
		0.025,0.05% cream	20,45 gm
		0.1% cream	20 gm
		0.01%,0.025% gel	15,45 gm

Types:
C = cream
G = gel
L = lotion
O = ointment
S = solution
ST = stick

Most preparations below are used bid.

*Sulfo-Lac, sulfurated lime (hot compresses),
 Vlemasque are used 15–20 minutes daily.

**Night Cast is used 30 minutes daily.

Preparation	Type	Size
Acno	L	120 ml
Acnomel	C	30 gm
Acnotex	L	60 ml
Bensulfoid	L	60 ml
Clearasil adult	C	18 gm
	ST	3.75 gm
Clinique anti-acne	C	
Cuticura	O	52.5 gm
Finac	L	60 ml
Fostex	C	120 gm
Fostril	L	30 ml
Komed	L	52.5 ml
Liquimat (acne cover-up)	L	45 ml
Lotio Alsulfa	L	120 ml
**Night Cast Formula R (mask)	L	120 ml
**Night Cast Formula S (mask)	L	120 ml
RA Lotion	L	120,240,480 ml
Rezamid	L	60 ml
SAStid plain	C	75 gm
Seale's lotion	L	60,120,240,480 ml
Sebasorb	L	60 ml
Rx Sulfacet R	L	25 ml
Sulforcin	L	120 ml
Sulfurated lime (Vleminckx soln)	L	480 ml
*Sulpho-Lac	C	30,52.5 gm
Therac	L	60 ml
Transact	G	30 gm
*Vlemasque (mask)	L	120 ml
Xerac	G	45 gm
Rx Xerac-AC	S	35,60 ml

EFFECTS OF INDIVIDUAL INGREDIENTS

Antibacterial

Antifungal
Antiparasitic
Antipruritic
Drying Agent
Keratolytic

Ingredients

A = alcohol	R = resorcinol
AC = acetone	S = sulfur
AL = aluminum chloride	SA = salicylic acid
C = calamine	SS = sodium sulfacetamide
L4 = laureth-4	ST = sodium thiosulfate
MBC = methylbenzethonium Cl	T = thymol
MC = menthol, camphor	VS = Vleminckx solution
MS = methyl salicylate	(sulfurated lime)
OX = oxyquinolone	ZO = zinc oxide
P = phenol	ZS = zinc sulfate

S	SA	R	A	ST	L4	Other
3%	2%					
8%		2%	11%			
8%	2.55%		22%			AC,MBC
6%			12%			5% MS, 0.5% T, 6% ZO
8%		1%				
5%	1%					
0.5% (precip. sulfur)						0.05% OX, 0.1% P
2%			8%			MBC
2%	2%					
2%					6%	
	2%		25%	8%		MC
5%			22%			
5%						
8%		2%				
4%	1.5%					
		3%	43%			6% C, 6% Starch
5%		2%	28.5%			
1.6%	1.6%					
6.4%						AC, Bentonite, ZO
2%	2%					10% Attapulgite
5%						10% SS
5%			11.65%			
						VS
5%						53% VS, 27% ZS
4%	2.35%					
2%			40%		6%	
						6% VS
4%			44%			
						6.25% AL (for folliculitis)
*		*	*	*		AC,MBC,OX,P,SS,T,ZO, AL,VS,ZS
*			*	*		MBC,T,VS
*					*	VS
	*					MC,P
			*			AL,C,Starch,ZS,ZO
*	*	*			*	VS

(A) Most are possible sensitizers (pramoxine less than most others).
(B) Not useful on intact epidermis with stratum corneum.
(C) Useful on oral mucosa, anogenital mucosa.
(D) Not effective for sunburn (except 10–20% benzocaine).
(E) Pramoxine effective in some dermatoses as an antipruritic when combined with HC.

Brand Name	Generic
GENERAL PRODUCTS:	
AeroCaine	Benzocaine/BCL
AeroTherm	Benzocaine/BCL
Americaine	Benzocaine
Bactine	Lidocaine
Bicozene	Benzocaine
Butesin Picrate	Butamben picrate
Calamatum	Benzocaine/ZO/ calamine/camphor
Rx Cetacaine	Benzocaine/ 2% tetracaine/BCL/ 2% butamben picrate
Chiggerex	Benzocaine/M/camphor
Rx Corticaine	Dibucaine/1% HC
Rx Dermasone	Pramoxine/1% HC
Dermocaine	Tetracaine
Dermoplast	Benzocaine
Rx Epifoam	Pramoxine/1% HC
Foille	Benzocaine
Rx Lida-Mantle-HC	Lidocaine/0.5% HC
Medicone Derma	Benzocaine/M/I/ZO
Rx Medicone Derma HC	(above)+1% HC
Medicone Dressing	Benzocaine/ZO/M/CLO
Medi-Quik	Lidocaine/BCL
Nupercainal	Dibucaine
Pontocaine	Tetracaine
PrameGel	Pramoxine/0.5% M
Rx Pramosone	Pramoxine/0.5% HC
	Pramoxine/1% HC
	Pramoxine/2.5% HC
Prax	Pramoxine
Rhulicaine	Benzocaine/M/tricolosan
Soft 'N Soothe	Benzocaine/M
Solarcaine	Benzocaine/triclosan
Sting-Kill	Benzocaine/M
Tronothane	Pramoxine
Unguentine	Benzocaine

BCL = benzalkonium Cl
CLO = cod liver oil
HC = hydrocortisone
I = icthammol
M = menthol
ZO = zinc oxide

Preparation	Size	Action or Dosage
13.6% spray	15,75 gm	< 1 hr
13.6% spray	150 gm	< 1 hr
20% ointment (burns)	22.5 gm	< 1 hr
20% spray	20,60,120 ml	
2.5% spray	90 ml	< 1 hr
2.5% liquid	60,120,480 ml	
6% cream	30 gm	< 1 hr
1% ointment	30 gm	
3% lotion (+phenol)	112.5 ml	< 1 hr
Ointment (+phenol)	45 gm	
1.05% spray (+M)	90 gm	
14% gel	29 gm	< 1 hr
14% liquid	56 ml	
14% ointment	37 gm	
14% spray	56 gm	
Ointment	52.5 gm	< 1 hr
0.5% cream	30 gm	2–4 hours, potent
1% cream	120 gm	2–4 hours
2% gel	60 gm	< 1 hr
20% spray/0.5% M	85 gm	< 1 hr
8% lotion	90 ml	
1% foam aerosol	10 gm	2–4 hours
2% spray	97.5,105 gm	< 1 hr
2% ointment	30 gm	
3% cream	30 gm	< 1 hr
2% ointment	30 gm	< 1 hr
2% ointment	7,20 gm	< 1 hr
0.5% ointment	30 gm	< 1 hr
Spray	90 ml	< 1 hr
0.5% cream	45 gm	2–4 hours, potent
1% ointment	30,60 gm	
1% cream	30 gm	< 1 hr
0.5% ointment	30 gm	
1% gel	118 gm	2–4 hours
1% lotion	60,120,240 ml	2–4 hours
1% cream	30,480 gm	
1% lotion	60,120,240 ml	2–4 hours
1% cream, ointment	30,120,480 gm	
1% lotion	60,120 ml	2–4 hours
1% cream, ointment	30,120,480 gm	
1% cream	30,120,480 gm	2–4 hours
1% lotion	15,120,240 ml	
20% spray	120 gm	< 1 hr
1% cream	50 gm	< 1 hr
20% spray	105 gm	< 1 hr
1% cream	30,60 gm	
0.5% lotion	90,180 ml	
18.9% swabs	0.5,14 ml	< 1 hr
1% cream	30 gm	2–4 hours
3% spray	90 gm	< 1 hr

HC = hydrocortisone
PCM = parachlorometaxylenol

Brand Name	Generic
GENERAL PRODUCTS (CONTINUED):	
Unguentine Plus	Benzocaine/phenol/PCM
Rx Vio-Pramasone	Pramoxine/Iodo
Rx Zone-A	Pramoxine/1% HC
Rx Zone-A Forte	Pramoxine/2.5% HC
ORAL AND NASAL PRODUCTS:	
Rx Americaine	Benzocaine
Benzodent	Benzocaine
CEPASTAT	Phenol
Rx Cetacaine	Benzocaine/ 2% tetracaine
Chloraseptic	Phenol
Rx Dyclone	Dyclonine HCl
Hurricaine	Benzocaine
Kank-a	Benzocaine
Orabase with Benzocaine	Benzocaine
Orajel regular maximum strength	Benzocaine
Orajel/d	Benzocaine
Pontocaine	Tetracaine
Rid-A-Pain	Benzocaine
Rx Xylocaine	Lidocaine
(Note: 2.5% ointment is OTC)	
PERIANAL PRODUCTS:	
Americaine	Benzocaine
Rx Analpram HC	Pramoxine/1% HC
Anusol	Pramoxine/ZO
Medicone rectal ointment	Benzocaine/castor oil/ M/ZO/hydroxyquinoline
Pazo Hemorrhoid	Benzocaine/ephedrine/ camphor/ZO
Rx Proctocream	Pramoxine/1% HC
Proctofoam	Pramoxine
Rx Proctofoam-HC	Pramoxine/1% HC
Tronolane	Pramoxine
SURGICAL TOPICAL ANESTHETIC SPRAYS:	
Rx Ethyl Chloride	Ethyl chloride
Rx Fluori-Methane	Dichlordifluoromethane 15%, Trichlormonofluoromethane 85%
Rx Fluoro-Ethyl spray	DCTF 75%, ethyl chloride 25%
Rx Gebauer's 114 spray	Dichlorotetrafluoroethane (DCTF)

Iodo = iodochlorhydroxyquin
ZO = zinc oxide

Preparations	Sizes	Action or Dosage
2% cream	30 gm	< 1 hr
Cream	30 gm	2–4 hours
1% lotion	60 ml	2–4 hours
1% cream	30 gm	
1% lotion	60 ml	2–4 hours
20% gel	30 gm	< 1 hr
20% ointment	7.5,30 gm	< 1 hr
0.73,1.45% lozenges	18/box	< 1 hr
14% spray	56 gm	< 1 hr
14% solution	56 ml	
14% ointment	37 gm	
14% gel	29 gm	
1.4% spray	180,360 ml	< 1 hr
32.5 mg lozenges	18,36/box	
0.5, 1% solution	30 ml	< 1 hr
20% gel	30 gm	< 1 hr
20% solution	30 ml	
20% spray	60 gm	
5% liquid	4.5 ml	< 1 hr
20% paste	5,15 gm	< 1 hr
10% gel	5,10 gm	< 1 hr
20% gel	5,10 gm	
10% gel	10 gm	< 1 hr
2% solution	30,120 ml	< 1 hr
0.5% solution	15,60 ml	
10% gel	10 gm	< 1 hr
4% solution	50 ml	< 1 hr
2% viscous solution	20,100,450 ml	
10% oral spray	60 ml	
2.5,5% ointment	35 gm	
5% flavored ointment	3.5,35 gm	
20% ointment (hemorrhoids)	30 gm	< 1 hr
1% cream	30 gm	2–4 hours
1% ointment	30,60 gm	2–4 hours
2% ointment	45 gm	< 1 hr
0.8% ointment	30,60 gm	< 1 hr
1% cream	30 gm	2–4 hours
1% foam aerosol	15 gm	2–4 hours
1% foam aerosol	10 gm	2–4 hours
1% cream	30,60 gm	2–4 hours
	120 gm	
	120 gm	
	270 gm	
	240 gm	

Problem/Organism
Acne
Actinomyces
Anthrax
Bacteroides
Borrelia recurrentis
Brucella
Calymmatobacterium granulomatis
Campylobacter
Cellulitis (extremity)
Cellulitis (facial)
Cellulitis (facial, child)
Clostridia
Erythrasma
Gram-negative folliculitis
Haemophilus influenzae (non-life threatening)
Human bite
Impetigo
Listeria monocytogenes
Lyme disease
Meningococcus
Mycoplasma
Nocardia
Pasteurella multocida
Perioral dermatitis
Pneumococcus
Rickettsia
Shigella
Staphylococcus (See: Impetigo)
Streptococcus

Regimen for STD
Chancroid
Chlamydia
Gonorrhea (In most cases treat also for *Chlamydia*)
Lymphogranuloma venereum
NGU
Syphilis (< 1 yr)
Syphilis (> 1 yr) except neurosyphilis

Modified from Sanford JP. Guide to antimicrobial therapy.
West Bethesda, MD: Jay P. Sanford, M.D., 1988.

Amox/PC = amoxicillin/potassium clavulanate   Clox = cloxacillin
Diclox = dicloxicillin   DS = double strength   TCN = Tetracycline
TMP/SMX = trimethoprim/sulfamethoxazole

First Choice	Second Choice
Erythromycin, TCN, and related drugs	
Ampicillin or penicillin	TCN
Penicillin	TCN, Erythromycin
Metronidazole	Clindamycin
TCN	Erythromycin
TCN	TMP/SMX
TCN	TMP/SMX
Erythromycin	Ciprofloxacin
Penicillin	Erythromycin
Clox, diclox, nafcillin, oxacillin	Cephalosporin
IV antibiotics	Amox/PC
Penicillin	TCN
Erythromycin	Topical agents
Ampicillin, TMP/SMX	—
Amox/PC	Cefaclor, TMP/SMX
Amox/PC	—
Clox, diclox, nafcillin, oxacillin	Erythromycin
Ampicillin	TMP/SMX
TCN	Penicillin
Penicillin	Chloramphenicol
Erythromycin	TCN
Sulfonamide	Minocycline
Penicillin	TCN
TCN	Erythromycin, Minocycline
Penicillin	Erythromycin
TCN	Chloramphenicol
TMP/SMX	Ampicillin
Penicillin	Erythromycin

First Choice	Second Choice
Erythromycin 500 qid × 7d or Ceftriaxone 250 IM	TMP/SMX DS bid × 7d or Amox/PC tid × 7d
TCN 500 qid × 7d	Erythromycin 500 qid × 7d
Ceftriaxone 250 IM + TCN 500 qid × 7d or Doxycycline 100 mg bid × 7d	Spectinomycin 2 gm IM + TCN 500 qid × 7d or Doxycycline 100 bid × 7d
TCN 500 qid × 21d	Erythromycin 500 qid × 21d or Doxycycline 100 bid × 21d
TCN 500 qid × 7d	Erythromycin 500 qid × 7d
Benzathine Pen G 2.4 million units IM	TCN 500 qid × 15d or Erythromycin 500 qid × 15d
Same but repeat weekly × 3	Same but give 30-day course

Generic	Brand Name
Rx Amoxicillin	Amoxil, Trimox Polymox, Wymox
Rx Amoxicillin + potassium clavulanate	Augmentin
Rx Ampicillin	Amcill, Omnipen, Polycillin, Principen
Rx Bacampicillin	Spectrobid
Rx Cefaclor	Ceclor
Rx Cefadroxil	Duricef, Ultracef
Rx Cefuroxime	Ceftin
Rx Cephalexin	Keflet, Keftab Keflex
Rx Cephradine	Anspor, Velosef
Rx Chloramphenicol	Chloromycetin
Rx Ciprofloxacin	Cipro
Rx Clindamycin	Cleocin
Rx Cloxacillin	Cloxapen, Tegopen
Rx Cyclacillin	Cyclapen-W
Rx Demeclocycline	Declomycin
Rx Dicloxicillin	Dynapen Pathocil
Rx Doxycycline	Vibramycin Doryx
Rx Erythromycin (enteric coated)	ERYC, ERY-Tab, E-Mycin, Ilotycin, Robimycin ERY-Tab, E-Mycin, PCE Dispertabs ERY-Tab
Rx Erythromycin (stearate)	Erythocin Stearate, Wyamycin-S
Rx Erythromycin (estolate)	Ilosone
Rx Erythromycin (ethylsuccinate)	EES (also E-Mycin E, Pediamycin, Wyamycin E suspensions)

*Tetracycline, erythromycin stearate, generic erythromycin (no enteric coating), and Penicillin V should be taken with water on an empty stomach. Tetracycline, erythromycin, doxycline, and minocycline may be tapered to a dose lower than listed to maintain chronic acne patients. Tetracycline suspension diluted to 250 mg/60 ml water makes an effective antibiotic mouthwash.

+Augmentin: Do not use two 250 mg pills to equal 500 mg, since clavulanic acid toxicity may result.

Note: Consult manufacturer's prescribing information and the medical literature for exact dosage in various dermatologic conditions.

Preparation	Dose (mg)
125,250,500 mg	250 tid
250,500 mg	
125,250,500 mg	250–500 tid+
250,500 mg	250–500 q6h
400 mg	400–800 bid
250,500 mg	250–500 tid
500,1000 mg	1–2 gm/24 h (qd-bid)
125,250,500 mg	250–500 bid
250,500 mg	250–500 q6h
250,500,1000 mg	
250,500 mg	250–500 q6h
250 mg	250–750 q6h
250,500,750 mg	250–750 bid
75,150,300 mg	150–450 q6h
250,500 mg	250–500 q6h
250,500 mg	250–500 qid
150,300 mg	150 qid or 300 bid
125,250,500 mg	125–500 q6h
250,500 mg	
50,100 mg	100–200/24h (qd-bid)*
100 mg	
250 mg	250–500 q6h*
333 mg	
500 mg	
250,500 mg	250–500 qid*
125,250,500 mg	250–500 qid*
250,400 mg	400–1000 qid*

DS = double strength

Generic	Brand Names
Rx Methacycline	Rondomycin
Rx Minocycline	Minocin
Rx Nafcillin	Unipen
Rx Norfloxicin	Noroxin
Rx Oxacillin	Bactocill, Prostaphlin
Rx Oxytetracycline	Terramycin
Rx Penicillin V	Betapen-VK, Ledercillin-VK, Pen-Vee K, Veetids VCillin K
Rx Rifampin	Rifadin Rimactane
Rx Sulfamethoxazole	Gantanol, Gantanol DS
Rx Sulfisoxazole	Gantrisin
Rx Tetracycline	Panmycin Achromycin V, Sumycin
Rx Trimethoprim, sulfamethoxazole	Bactrim, Cotrim, Septra Bactrim DS, Cotrim DS, Septra DS

*Tetracycline, erythromycin stearate, generic erythromycin (no enteric coating), and Penicillin V should be taken with water on an empty stomach. Tetracycline, erythromycin, doxycycline, and minocycline may be tapered to a dose lower than listed to maintain chronic acne patients. Tetracycline suspension diluted to 250 mg/60 ml water makes an effective antibiotic mouthwash.

Note: Consult manufacturer's prescribing information and the medical literature for exact dosage in various dermatologic conditions.

Preparation	Dose (mg)
150,300 mg	150 q6h
50,100 mg	200/24h* (bid-qid)
250,500 mg	250–1000 q4–6h
400 mg	400 bid
250,500 mg	500 q4–6h
250 mg	250–500 qid
250,500 mg	250–500 qid*
125,250,500 mg	
150,300 mg	600 qd
300 mg	
500 mg	1000 bid-tid
1000 mg	
500 mg	1000 qid–6x/d
250 mg	250–500 qid*
250,500 mg	
400/80 mg	2 bid
800/160 mg	1 bid

*Avoid usage in children < 8 years old. May cause permanent tooth discoloration.

Generic	Brand Name	Size
Rx Amoxicillin	Amoxil	80,100,150 ml
	Polymox	80,100,150 ml
	Trimox	80,100,150 ml
	Wymox	100,150 ml
	Wymox	80,100,150 ml
Rx Amoxicillin + potassium clavulonate	Augmentin	75,150 ml
Rx Ampicillin	Amcill	100,200 ml
	Omnipen	100,150,200 ml
	Polycillin	80,100,150,200 ml
	Polycillin	100 ml
	Principen	100,150,200 ml
Rx Bacampicillin	Spectrobid	70,100 ml
Rx Cefaclor	Ceclor	75,150 ml
		50,100 ml
Rx Cefadroxil	Duricef	50,100 ml
	Duricef	100 ml
	Ultracef	50,100 ml
Rx Cephalexin	Keflex	60,100,200 ml
	Keflex	100,200 ml
Rx Cephradine	Anspor	100 ml
	Velosef	100,200 ml
Rx Chloramphenicol	Chloromycetin	60 ml
Rx Cloxacillin	Tegopen	100,200 ml
Rx Cyclacillin	Cyclapen-W	100,150,200 ml
Rx Dicloxicillin	Dynapen	80,100,200 ml
	Pathocil	100 ml
Rx Doxycycline	Vibramycin	60 ml
Rx Erythromycin-ethylsuccinate	EES	60,100,200,480 ml
	EES-400	100,480 ml
	E-Mycin E	500 ml
	Pediamycin	50 ml
	Pediamycin	100,150,480 ml
	Pediamycin	480 ml
	Wyamycin E	480 ml
Rx Minocycline	Minocin	60 ml
Rx Nafcillin	Unipen	100 ml
Rx Oxacillin	Prostaphlin	100 ml
Rx Penicillin V	Betapen-VK	100,200 ml
	Ledercillin-VK	100,150,200 ml
	Pen Vee K	100,200 ml
	Pen Vee K	100,150,200 ml
	VCillin K	100,150,200 ml
	Veetids	100,200 ml
Rx Tetracycline*	Achromycin-V	480 ml
	Sumycin	480 ml
Rx Trimethoprim-sulfamethoxazole	Bactrim	100,480 ml
	Cotrim	480 ml
	Septra	100,150,200,480 ml

Preparation	Dose (up to 40 kg)
125 or 250 mg/5 ml	20–40
125 or 250 mg/5 ml	mg/kg/d (q8h)
125 or 250 mg/5 ml	
125 mg/5 ml	
250 mg/5 ml	
125 or 250 mg/5 ml	20–40 mg/kg/d
125 or 250 mg/5 ml	50–100
125 or 250mg/5 ml	mg/kg/d (q6h)
125 or 250 mg/5 ml	(up to 20 kg)
500 mg/5 ml	
125 or 250 mg/5 ml	
125 mg/5 ml	25–50 mg/kg/d (q12h)
125 or 250 mg/5 ml	20–40
187 or 375 mg/5 ml	mg/kg/d (q8h)
125 or 250 mg/5 ml	30 mg/kg/d (q12h)
500 mg/5 ml	
125 or 250 mg/5 ml	
125 mg/5 ml	25–50 mg/kg/d (q6h)
250mg/5 ml	
125 or 250 mg/5 ml	25–100
125 or 250 mg/5 ml	mg/kg/d (bid–qid)
150 mg/5 ml	50 mg/kg/d (q6h)
125 mg/5 ml	50 mg/kg/d (q6h)
125 or 250 mg/5 ml	50–100 mg/kg/d (q6h)
62.5 mg/5ml	12.5–50
62.5 mg/5 ml	mg/kg/d (q6h)
25 mg/5 ml	5 mg/kg/d (bid)
200 mg/5 ml	30–100
400 mg/5 ml	mg/kg/d (q6h)
200 or 400 mg/5 ml	
100 mg/2.5 ml	
200 mg/5 ml	
400 mg/5 ml	
200 or 400 mg/5 ml	
50 mg/5 ml	4 mg/kg then
	2 mg/kg q12h
250 mg/5 ml	25–50 mg/kg/d (q6h)
250 mg/5 ml	50 mg/kg/d (q6h)
125 or 250 mg/5 ml	50 mg/kg/d
125 or 250 mg/5 ml	(q6h–q8h)
125 mg/5 ml	
250 mg/5 ml	
125 or 250 mg/5 ml	
125 or 250 mg/5 ml	
125 mg/5 ml	25–50 mg/kg/d (q6h)
125 mg/5 ml	
	0.5ml/kg q12h

(A) Useful primarily as prophylaxis (for
pyodermas: use oral antibiotics).
(B) For open wounds: bacitracin, garamycin, polymyxin,
povidone (small wounds), silver sulfadiazene.
(C) For *Staphylococcus:* mupirocin, neomycin.
(D) For other Gram-positive: bacitracin, gramicidin.

Note: Bac = bacitracin   HC = hydrocortisone   Neo = neomycin
      Iodo = iodochlorhydroxyquin   Poly = polymyxin

Brand Name	Type	Generic Name	Preparation
Achromycin	ointment	3% Tetracycline	15,30 gm
Aureomycin	ointment	3% Chlortetracycline	15,30 gm
Baciguent	ointment	Bacitracin	15,30 gm
Bactine Triple Antibiotic	ointment	Poly/neo/bac	15 gm
Rx Bactroban	ointment	2% Mupirocin	15 gm
Betadine	ointment	Povidone	30,480, 2400 gm
Rx Caquin	cream	3% Iodo/1% HC	20 gm
Rx Chloromycetin	cream	1% chloramphenicol	30 gm
Rx Cordran-N	cream	Neo/flurandrenolide	15,30,60 gm
	ointment		15,30,60 gm
Rx Cortin	cream	3% Iodo/1% HC	20 gm
Rx Cortisporin	cream	Poly/neo/0.5% HC	7.5 gm
	ointment	Poly/neo/bac/1% HC	15 gm
Rx Furacin	cream	0.2% nitrofurazone	28 gm
	ointment		28,56,454 gm
Rx Garamycin	cr, oint	0.1% gentamicin	15 gm
Rx G-myticin	cr, oint	0.1% gentamicin	15 gm
Iodex	ointment	Povidone	30,435 gm
Myciguent	cream	0.5% Neo	15 gm
	ointment		15,30,120 gm
Mycitracin	ointment	Poly/neo/bac	15,30 gm
Rx Neo-Cort-Dome	cream	Neo/0.5% HC	15 gm
Rx Neo Cortef	cream	Neo/1% HC	20 gm
	ointment	Neo/0.5% HC	20 gm
		Neo/1% HC	5,20 gm
		Neo/2.5% HC	5,20 gm

ANTIBIOTICS, TOPICAL (See also: Acne Medications)

(E) For Gram-negative: gentamycin (*Pseudomonas* resistance
    common), neomycin (except *Pseudomonas*), polymyxin
    (except *Proteus, Serratia*), silver sulfadiazene.
(F) For burns: mafenide (penetrates eschar, often painful,
    common sensitizer), nitrofurazone (common sensitizer),
    silver nitrate (see Wet Dressings), silver sulfadiazene.
(G) For bacteria and fungus: iodochlorhydroxyquin,
    iodoquinone, povidone.

cr = cream
oint = ointment
lotn = lotion
soln = solution

Brand Name	Type	Generic Name	Preparation
Rx Neodecadron	cream	Neo/0.1% dexamethasone	15,30 gm
Rx Neo-Medrol	ointment	Neo/1%, 0.25% methylprednisolone	30 gm
Neosporin	cream	Poly/neo	15 gm
	ointment	Poly/neo/bac	15,30 gm
Rx Neo-Synalar	cream	Neo/0.025% fluocinolone	15,30,60 gm
Rx Nitrofurazone	soln	0.2% nitrofurazone	480,3840 ml
Rx Pedi-Cort-V	cream	3% Iodo/1% HC	20 gm
Polysporin	ointment	Poly/bac	15,30 gm
	powder		10 gm
	spray		90 gm
Rx Racet	cream	3% Iodo/0.5% HC	15,30 gm
Rx Silvadene	cream	1% silver sulfadiazene	20,50,85 400,1000 gm
Spectrocin	ointment	Neo/gramicidin	15,30 gm
Rx Sulfamylon	cream	Mafenide acetate	60,120,435 gm
Terramycin	ointment	Oxytetracycline	15,30 gm
Terramycin/ Polymyxin	ointment powder	Oxytetracycline/poly	30,150 gm 30 gm
Rx UAD	cream lotion	3% Iodo/1% HC	15 gm 120 ml
Vioform cream,	oint	3% Iodo	30 gm
Rx Vioform HC	lotion	3% Iodo/1% HC	15 ml
	cream		5,20 gm
	ointment		20 gm
Rx Vioform HC mild	cream	3% Iodo/0.5% HC	15,30 gm
	ointment		30 gm
Rx Vytone	cream	Iodoquinol/0.5%, 1% HC	30 gm

(Including antileprosy agents and antimalarials)
(Isotretinoin: See Acne Medications, Oral)

      5FU = 5 fluorouracil

1. 5FU: To decrease inflammation, can add
   0.5% triamcinolone cream.
2. 5FU: For resistant cases, can add 0.05% tretinoin cream.
3. Clofazimine is designed for use as part of a multiple drug
   regimen for leprosy.

	Brand Name	Generic
Rx	Aralen	Chloroquine**
Rx	Atabrine	Quinicrine
Rx	Azulfidine	Sulfasalazine
Rx	Chloroquine	Chloroquine**
Rx	Colchicine	Colchicine
Rx	Cytoxan	Cyclophosphamide
Rx	Dapsone	Dapsone**
Rx	Efudex	5FU 5% cream
		5FU 2%, 5% solution
Rx	Fluoroplex	5FU 1% cream
		5FU 1% solution
Rx	Hydrea	Hydroxyurea
Rx	Imuran	Azothioprine
Rx	Intron A	Alpha 2b interferon
Rx	Lamprene	Clofazimine
Rx	Leukeran	Chlorambucil
Rx	Mustargen	Nitrogen mustard
Rx	Plaquenil	Hydroxychloroquine**
Rx	Rheumatrex	Methotrexate**
Rx	Roferon-A	Alpha 2a interferon
Rx	Sandimmune	Cyclosporine**
Rx	Sulfapyridine	Sulfapyridine**
Rx	Tegison	Etretinate**
Rx	Thioguanine	Thioguanine

*Please consult product inserts and the medical literature for the specific indications
 and dosages of these drugs in the treatment of individual dermatologic conditions.

**DETAILED INFORMATION ON CHLOROQUINE, CYCLOSPORINE, DAPSONE,
ETRETINATE, HYDROXYCHLOROQUINE, METHOTREXATE, AND SULFAPYRIDINE
FOLLOWS ON THE NEXT TEN PAGES.

ANTICANCER DRUGS AND IMMUNOMODULATORS   **31**
(Including antileprosy agents and antimalarials)
(Isotretinoin: See Acne Medications, Oral)

Preparation	Dose*
500 mg (=300 mg base)	250–500 mg/d
100 mg	200–800 mg/d
500 mg, 250 mg/5 ml	1–4 gm/d (qid)
250 mg (=150 mg base)	250–500 mg/d
0.6 mg	0.6–1.8 mg/d (qd-tid)
25,50,100,200,500,1000,2000 mg	1–5 mg/kg/d
25,100 mg	50–300 mg/d (qd-bid)
25 gm	bid X 2-4 wks
10 ml	
30 gm	bid X 2-6 wks
30 ml	
500 mg	20-30 mg/kg/d or 80 mg/kg/3d
50,100 mg	1-3 mg/kg/d
3,5,10,25,50 $\times$ 10^6 unit vials	2×10^6 IU/m^2 3$\times$/wk
50,100 mg	50-100 mg/d
2 mg	0.1–0.2 mg/kg/d
10 mg vials	0.4 mg/kg/d
200 mg	200–400 mg/d (qd-bid)
2.5 mg	2.5 mg q12h $\times$ 3 each week
3,18,36 $\times$ 10^6 unit vials	3×10^6 units qod-qd
100 mg/ml	3–14 mg/kg/d
500 mg	1–4 gm/d (qid)
10,25 mg	0.5–1.5 mg/kg/d (bid)
40 mg	2–3 mg/kg/d

CHLOROQUINE (Aralen)
HYDROXYCHLOROQUINE (Plaquenil)

DOSAGE:

(1) Lupus Erythematosus: 400 mg/d for several weeks then try to reduce to 200 mg/d.

(2) Rheumatoid Arthritis: 400–600 mg/d.

(3) Porphyria Cutanea Tarda: 100–200 mg twice weekly for 2 weeks then 3x/wk until clinical response adequate.

LAB TESTS:

(1) Ophthalmic exam: Baseline and q3–6 mos.

(2) Complete blood count (CBC): Baseline and periodically (some physicians recommend CBC qmo x3 then q4–6 mos).

(3) Other labs: G6PD (optional). Some physicians follow BUN, creatinine, liver function tests.

CONTRAINDICATIONS:

(1) Retinal disease.

(2) Pregnancy.

(3) Use extreme caution in children (plaquenil has caused some fatalities in children).

(4) Use extreme caution with liver disease, alcoholism, or in patients taking other hepatotoxic drugs.

(5) Psoriasis: Antimalarials often cause psoriasis to flare.

SIDE EFFECTS:

(1) Ocular
    (a) Retinopathy: Dose related (usually after total dose of 200 gm and less likely with lower doses such as chloroquine 250 mg/d, hydroxychloroquine 200 mg/d). Irreversible. May be more common with chloroquine than hydroxychloroquine. May be symptomatic.
    (b) Corneal opacities (reversible).
    (c) Blurred or double vision (temporary).

(2) Hematologic
    (a) Agranulocytosis, aplastic anemia: both are rare and reversible. Usually in first 3 months of treatment.
    (b) Hemolysis (G6PD deficient patients).

(3) Cutaneous
    (a) Blue-black pigmentation of skin, nail beds, mucous membranes.
    (b) Bleaching of hair.
    (c) Lichenoid dermatitis, exfoliative erythroderma.

(4) Other
    (a) Nausea, vomiting, diarrhea, headache, pruritus, sweating.
    (b) Myopathy, neuropathy: Check muscle strength and deep tendon reflexes periodically.
    (c) Toxic psychosis (rare).

HOW SUPPLIED:

(1) Chloroquine: 250 mg (generic), 500 mg (Aralen).

(2) Hydroxychloroquine: 200 mg (Plaquenil).

CYCLOSPORINE (Sandimmune)

DOSAGE (psoriasis):

(1) Dosages for psoriasis have not been standardized and have ranged from 1 mg/kg/d to 15 mg/kg/d.

(2) Current recommendations are to start at 5 mg/kg/d and reduce, if possible, according to clinical response.

LAB TESTS:

(1) Baseline studies should include CBC, differential, platelets, BUN, creatinine, liver function tests, and chemistry panel.

(2) As a minimum, renal function tests, liver function tests, and serum potassium should also be followed during treatment. CBC and chemistry panel may also be followed.

(3) Side effects can be minimized by keeping trough blood levels (whole blood radioimmunoassay) < 250 ng/ml.

(4) Some physicians also obtain creatinine clearance and pregnancy tests.

INTERACTIONS:

(1) Drugs increasing cyclosporine levels include erythromycin, high-dose methylprednisolone, ketoconazole, and amphotericin B.

(2) Drugs lowering cyclosporine levels include rifampin, phenytoin, and phenobarbitol.

(3) Avoid potassium-sparing diuretics and nephrotoxic drugs.

SIDE EFFECTS:

(1) Nephrotoxicity: Usually reversible with dosage reduction. If serum creatinine increases by 30% over baseline, reduce cyclosporine dose by 25%.

(2) Hepatoxicity: Reversible with dosage reduction.

(3) Hypertension: Follow blood pressure.

(4) Tremor, headaches, paresthesias, rarely seizures.

(5) Hypertrichosis (common).

(6) Gingival hyperplasia.

(7) Increased serum potassium possible. Occasionally seen are increased uric acid, triglycerides or cholesterol, anemia, decreased serum magnesium, or platelets.

(8) Other side effects include nausea, vomiting, diarrhea, increased blood clotting, bone marrow suppression, epidermal cysts, acne, folliculitis, and sebaceous hyperplasia.

(9) Increased incidence of infections (commonly viral).

(10) There may possibly be an increased incidence of lymphoma with cyclosporine treatment.

HOW SUPPLIED:

100 mg/ml (50 ml bottle)

ETRETINATE (Tegison)

DOSAGE:

(1) Initial: 0.5–1.0 mg/kg/d in two divided doses taken with food (0.25 mg/kg/d for erythrodermic psoriasis).

(2) Maximum: 1.5 mg/kg/d.

(3) Maintenance: 0.5–0.75 mg/kg/d often initiated after 8–16 weeks of therapy; however, therapy should be terminated when possible in patients with significant improvement.

LAB TESTS: Clinical visits suggested twice in first month, monthly for 6 months, then every 3 months.

(1) Pregnancy tests: Baseline, monthly during treatment, and for at least 1 year after treatment.
   (a) Two forms of contraception should be used during treatment and for at least 1 year after treatment.
   (b) Pregnancy should be avoided for at least 2 years after treatment.
   (c) Treatment should begin only in second or third day of next normal menstrual period following baseline labs.

(2) Triglycerides, cholesterol, HDL lipids: Baseline, each visit for 4 months, then every 3 months.
   (a) Obtain fasting levels (36 hours after last alcohol consumption).
   (b) Follow patients with personal or family history of diabetes mellitus, obesity, or heavy alcohol usage most closely since these patients are prone to development of elevated levels.

(3) SGOT, SGPT, LDH: Baseline, then each visit.

(4) X-rays:
   (a) Some physicians obtain annual lateral ankle radiographs.
   (b) Baseline and yearly for bone age (include knees) in children.

(5) Other: Some physicians monitor CBC with platelets, urinalysis (UA), blood chemistry, and glucose each visit for 1 year then every 6 months.

CONTRAINDICATIONS:

(1) Pregnancy, nursing mothers.

(2) Paraben allergy (capsules contain parabens).

INTERACTIONS:

(1) Vitamin A: May increase etretinate toxicity.

(2) Milk: Increases etretinate absorption.

HOW SUPPLIED:

10, 25 mg capsules.

ETRETINATE (Tegison) (continued)

SIDE EFFECTS:

(1) *Fetal abnormalities*

(2) *Pseudotumor cerebri (benign intracranial hypertension):*
    (a) Examine for papilledema if headache, nausea and vomiting, or visual changes ensue.
    (b) Stop treatment if papilledema present.

(3) *Hepatoxicity:*
    (a) Hepatitis (1.5%).
    (b) Elevated SGOT (18%), SGPT (23%), LDH (15%).
    (c) Stop treatment only if hepatoxicity suspected since mild changes in lab values often normalize despite continuing treatment.

(4) *Ocular changes:*
    (a) Various problems reported include corneal opacities, anterior subcapsular cataracts, decreased night vision, and decreased tolerance of contact lenses (also see chart below).
    (b) Stop treatment and get ophthalmologic examination if significant visual difficulties ensue.

Adverse Effects Reported in More than 1% of Patients

Body System	> 75%	50–75%
Mucocutaneous	Dry nose Chapped lips	Thirst Sore mouth
Dermatologic		Dry, itchy, or fragile skin
	Hair loss (mild)	Red, scaly face
	Palmoplantar peeling	Rash
Musculoskeletal	Hyperostosis	Bone/joint pain
Central Nervous System		
		Fatigue
Special Senses		
		Eye irritation
Gastrointestinal		
Other		
Laboratory		Elevated MCHC

(5) *Hyperostosis:*
   (a) After 60 months of treatment averaging 0.8 mg/kg/d, 84% of patients developed extraspinal tendon and ligament calcification (usually bilateral and multifocal), (ankles, pelvis, knees most commonly), (approximately 50% asymptomatic).

(6) *Lipids:*
   (a) Elevated triglycerides (45%), decreased HDL lipids (37%), increased cholesterol (16%).
   (b) Can often continue treatment and normalize values with weight loss, low fat diet, decreased alcohol consumption, and/or dosage reduction.
   (c) Stop therapy if triglyceride level exceeds 800 mg/dl.

25–50%	10–25%	1–10%*
	Chelitis	Dry mouth
Nosebleed	Sore tongue	Gingivitis
		Pyogenic granuloma
Bruising	Nail disorders	Bullae, hair problems, onycholysis, paronychia,
Photosensitivity	Skin peeling	sweat changes
Muscle cramps		Myalgia
		Dizziness
		Sensory changes
Headache	Fever	Lethargy, rigors
	Eye abnormalities	Dry eyes
	Conjunctivitis	Earache
Eye pain	Visual changes	Otitis externa
Abdominal pain		
Appetite changes	Nausea	Hepatitis
		Thrombosis, edema
		Dyspnea, malignancy
Elev. triglycerides	Elev. SGOT, SGPT,	Elev. BUN, creatinine,
Changes in electrolytes, calcium, phosphate, CBC	LDH, cholesterol Changes in UA, glucose	CPK, or bilirubin Changes in protein or albumin

Elev = elevated   *May not be related to etretinate therapy.

METHOTREXATE

DOSAGE (psoriasis):

(1) 2.5 to 5.0 mg every 12 hours for 3 doses weekly (or give in one large dose weekly).

(2) Can increase by 25 mg/wk if needed up to 30 mg/wk.

(3) Once maximum clinical effect achieved, taper to lowest effective dose.

LAB TESTS:

(1) Liver chemistry (AST, ALT, alkaline phosphatase, bilirubin, albumin). Baseline then q3–4 months. Obtain at least 1 week after last dose of methotrexate. If abnormal, stop drug and repeat in 1–2 weeks.

(2) BUN, creatinine: Baseline then q3–4 months.

(3) Complete blood count with differential and platelet count: Baseline then q1–4 wks.

(4) Urinalysis: Baseline then q3–4 months.

(5) Creatinine clearance: Baseline only. Some physicians repeat yearly. More accurate indicator than serum creatinine.

(6) Liver biopsy currently suggested, when feasible, at baseline or within first 4 months of treatment. Repeat every 1.5 gms cumulative dose (every 1.0 gms if patient has persisting abnormal liver chemistry or risk factors).

(7) Chest x-ray: Followed by some physicians.

CONTRAINDICATIONS:

(1) Pregnancy or nursing. Males and females must avoid conception during treatment (plus one additional menstrual cycle for women or three additional months for men).

(2) Significant liver disease or excessive alcohol use.

(3) Significant renal or pulmonary disease.

(4) Significant anemia, leukopenia, or thrombocytopenia.

(5) Active infectious disease.

(6) Immunodeficiency.

METHOTREXATE (continued)

INTERACTIONS:

(1) Drugs that may increase methotrexate toxicity include salicylates and nonsteroidal anti-inflammatory drugs (possibly severe interaction). Ethanol, sulfonamides, probenecid, penicillins, cephalosporins, colchicine, barbiturates, phenytoin, dipyridamole, and retinoids may also increase methotrexate toxicity.

(2) Drugs decreasing methotrexate toxicity include tetracycline, chloramphenicol, folic acid, and folinic acid.

SIDE EFFECTS (in doses used for psoriasis):

(1) General: Fever, chills.

(2) Skin: Pruritus, pain, urticaria, alopecia (mild, reversible), ecchymoses, ulcers.

(3) Blood: *Leukopenia, *thrombocytopenia, *anemia.

(4) Gastrointestinal: *Ulcerative stomatitis, nausea, anorexia. *Diarrhea, vomiting, enteritis less common.

(5) Hepatic: *Hepatotoxicity (incidence of cirrhosis low with total dose < 1.5 gm).

(6) Urogenital: Azotemia, hematuria, cystitis, defective gamete formation (reversible), *teratogenesis, menstrual changes, nephropathy.

(7) Neurologic: Headache, dizziness, drowsiness, blurred vision, depression.

(8) Respiratory: *Pneumonitis, *pulmonary fibrosis.

*Denotes potentially serious side effects that are most likely to require stopping methotrexate.

HOW SUPPLIED:

2.5 mg tablets

SULFAPYRIDINE AND DAPSONE

DOSAGE (Dapsone): Take with plenty of water to prevent renal precipitation.

(1) Dermatitis herpetiformis
   (a) 50–100 mg/d initially, increase to 100–300 mg/d over 2–3 weeks.
   (b) Some patients can be successfully tapered by 25 mg/week once controlled.
   (c) It takes 8 days to reach plateau blood levels. After continuous dosing, dapsone persists up to 35 days after discontinuing the drug.

(2) Leprosy
   (a) 100 mg/d for 20 years (borderline leprosy) or for life (lepromatous leprosy) plus:
   (b) Rifampin 600 mg/d × 2 years (and possibly clofazimine or ethionamide).

(3) Tuberculosis (bacteriologically negative)
   (a) 100 mg/d × 4–6 years plus:
   (b) Rifampin 600 mg/d × 6 months

DOSAGE (Sulfapyridine): Take with plenty of water to prevent renal precipitation.

(1) 1–6 gm/d (qid): Less effective than dapsone in most patients.

LAB TESTS:

(1) CBC with differential, platelet count, reticulocyte count: Baseline, weekly for 1 mo, monthly for 6 mos, then q6 mos.

(2) BUN, creatinine, urinalysis, liver function tests should also be monitored.

(3) G6PD: Baseline only.

INTERACTIONS:

(1) Probenecid increases dapsone half-life.

(2) Rifampin decreases dapsone half-life.

SULFAPYRIDINE AND DAPSONE (continued)

SIDE EFFECTS: (Most severe side effects occur within 3 months of treatment)

(1) Nausea, vomiting, headache, weakness, dizziness, fatigue, nervousness, shortness of breath (dose related, 20% incidence with dapsone, higher incidence with sulfapyridine).

(2) Hemolysis (dose related)
   (a) All patients have some hemolysis but not usually significant with dapsone at 100 mg/d.
   (b) Hematocrit can drop by 25% in 3-4 weeks with dapsone at 300 mg/d (faster with G6PD deficiency).
   (c) Fulminant hemolysis and acute tubular necrosis can occur during first week of treatment (more common in children and black patients).

(3) Methemoglobinemia (dose related)
   (a) All patients have some increase in methemoglobin.
   (b) Cyanosis occurs if 15% of total hemoglobin is methemoglobin.

(4) Leukopenia, agranulocytosis
   (a) Leukopenia occurs in 5% of patients on sulfapyridine (less with dapsone).
   (b) Agranulocytosis occurs in 0.01–0.1% of patients on dapsone; usually reversible but can be fatal.

(5) Hepatoxicity: Idiosyncratic, reversible, mostly seen with dapsone, can occur up to 9 mos after start of treatment.

(6) Nephrotoxicity: Due to renal precipitation, more common with sulfapyridine.

(7) Neuropathy: Distal motor neuropathy (mostly hands), slowly reversible, can occur up to years after start of treatment.

(8) Psychosis: Dose related.

(9) Cutaneous eruptions: Erythema multiforme, erythema nodosum, toxic epidermolytic necrolysis, and photosensitivity more common with sulfapyridine (10%).

(10) Hypersensitivity syndrome: Clinically similar to infectious mononucleosis—usually resolves but can be fatal.

(11) NOTE: Patients intolerant to dapsone may be able to take sulfapyridine without problems.

HOW SUPPLIED:

(1) Dapsone: 25, 100 mg

(2) Sulfapyridine: 500 mg

T = Tinea

Dermatophyte Infections

(1) Reported Cure Rates

(a)	Miconazole	> 90%	(T pedis)
(b)	Clotrimazole	60–100%	(Dermatophytes)
		20%	(T pedis 3 months after treatment
(c)	Ciclopirox	81–94%	(Dermatophytes, *Candida*)
(d)	Haloprogin	80%	(T pedis)
(e)	Tolnaftate	80%	(T pedis)
(f)	Undecylenic acid	< 50%	(T pedis)
(g)	Ketoconazole (oral)	83%	(*Resistant* dermatophytes)
		< 20%	(Onychomycosis, toenails)
(h)	Griseofulvin	53.3%	(T pedis, T manum)
		70%	(T pedis 3 months after treatment)
		32%	(*Resistant* dermatophytes)
		93.1%	(T capitis) (drug of choice)
		64.8%	(T cruris)
		56.9%	(Onychomycosis, fingernails) (drug of choice)
		16.7%	(Onychomycosis, toenails) (drug of choice) (If effective, topical agents may prevent reinfection)

(2) Castellani paint: Good for fissures, intertriginous areas.

(3) Aluminum chloride hexahydrate: Good for interdigital T pedis with bacterial involvement.

(4) Econazole, ketoconazole, naftifine, oxiconazole, sulconazole: Newer agents for resistant cases.

(5) Selenium sulfide: Helpful adjunct in treatment of T capitis.

(6) Antinea cream, Whitfield's ointment: Keratolytic, possible irritation, fungistatic.

(7) Other agents: Triacetin.

Pityrosporum

Ciclopirox, clotrimazole, econazole, haloprogin, ketoconazole (oral, topical), miconazole, selenium sulfide, sulconazole, Tinver Lotion, tolnaftate, zinc pyrithione (shampoo).

Candida

Amphotericin B (topical), ciclopirox, clotrimazole, econazole, haloprogin, ketoconazole (oral, topical), miconazole, nystatin.

Candida Vulvovaginitis

Butoconazole, clotrimazole, gentian violet, miconazole, nystatin, povidone, sulfanilamide, triple sulfa.

Antifungals with Gram-positive Antibacterial Activity

Castellani paint, clotrimazole, econazole, gentian violet, haloprogin, iodoquinol, iodochlorhydroxyquin, thymol (2–4% in absolute alcohol—very effective for paronchia).

Note: Griseofulvin: 150–200 mg ultra microsize = 250 mg microsize

Brand Name	Generic
Rx Ancobon	5 flucytosine
Rx Fulvicin-U/F*	Griseofulvin (micro)
Rx Fulvicin P/G*	Griseofulvin (ultra micro)
Rx Grifulvin V*	Griseofulvin (micro)
Rx Grifulvin V suspension*	Griseofulvin (micro)
Rx Grisactin*	Griseofulvin (micro)
Rx Grisactin Ultra*	Griseofulvin (ultra micro)
Rx Gris-PEG*	Griseofulvin (ultra micro)
Rx Mycelex troches	Clotrimazole
Rx Mycostatin suspension	Nystatin- 100,000 U/ml
Rx Mycostatin pastilles (troches)	Nystatin
Rx Mycostatin tablets	Nystatin
Rx Nilstat suspension	Nystatin 100,000 U/ml
Rx Nilstat tablets	Nystatin
Rx Nizoral+	Ketoconazole
Rx Nystex suspension	Nystatin- 100,000 U/ml
Rx SSKI solution	Potassium iodide 1 gm/ml

+*KETOCONAZOLE* (Delivered to skin in sweat)

(1) *Major side effects:*
Hepatotoxicity (1/10,000 patients, 60% in first 2 months, usually reversible, often presents with GI or abdominal complaints, rarely do fatal reactions occur). Anaphylaxis (rare).

(2) *Labs to follow:*
Liver function tests: Some physicians suggest obtaining every 2 weeks for 2 months then every month. Stop drug if persistently elevated.

(3) *Interactions:*
Rifampin, isoniazid, antihistamines, anticholinergics decrease ketoconazole effects. Ketoconazole increases effects of coumadin, cyclosporine A, and possibly oral hypoglycemics. Concomitant ketoconazole and phenytoin can alter levels of either drug.

Size	Adult Dose	Pediatric Dose
250,500 mg	50–150 mg/kg/d (q6°)	—
250,500 mg	500–1000 mg/qd	5 mg/lb/d
125,165,250,330 gm	330 mg (qd-bid)	3.3 mg/lb/d
250,500 mg	500–1000 mg qd	5 mg/lb/d
125 mg/5 cc	—	5 mg/lb/d
125,250,500 mg	500–1000 mg qd	5 mg/lb/d
125,250,330 mg	330 mg (qd-bid)	3.3 mg/lb/d
125,250 mg	375–750 mg qd	3.3 mg/lb/d
10 mg	5 times qd	—
5,60,473 ml	4–6 ml qid Swish and swallow	2 ml qid (infants)
200,000 U	1–2 qid-5×/d	—
500,000 U	1–2 tid	—
60,480 ml	4–6 ml qid Swish and swallow	2 ml qid (infants)
500,000 U	1–2 tid	—
200 mg	1–2 q A.M.	3.3–6.6 mg/kg/d (> 2 yrs)
60 ml	4–6 ml qid Swish and swallow	2 ml qid (infants)
30,240 ml	0.3–0.6 ml tid-qid	—

GRISEOFULVIN (Take with meals, fat increases absorption, sweat increases delivery to skin)

(1) *Major side effects:*
   Stop drug if granulocytopenia occurs.

(2) *Labs to follow:*
   CBC—Some physicians suggest obtaining every 2 weeks for 1 month then every 3 months.

(3) *Interactions:*
   Barbiturates decrease griseofulvin absorption. Griseofulvin increases the effects of alcohol and decreases the effects of coumadin. Griseofulvin possibly decreases the effectiveness of estrogen-containing oral contraceptives.

(4) *Contraindications:*
   Pregnancy, hepatocellular failure, acute intermittent porphyria.

(5) *Average Treatment Duration:* (T = tinea)
   T capitis (4–6 wks), T corporis (2–4 wks), T pedis (4–8 wks), onychomycosis (fingernails 4–6 mos, toenails 6–9 mos).

HC = hydrocortisone
Iodo = iodochlorhydroxyquin
T = Tinea

Exelderm: Apply qd
Nizoral: Apply qd
Oxystat: Apply qd
Others: Apply bid-tid

Brand Name	Generic	Size
Antinea	3% salicylic acid, 6% benzoic acid	30 gm
Rx Caquin	3% Iodo/1% HC	20 gm
Rx Cortin	3% Iodo/1% HC	20 gm
Cruex	Undecylenic acid	15 gm
Desenex	Undecylenic acid	15,30 gm
Enzactin	Triacetin	30 gm
Rx Exelderm	1% sulconazole	15,30,60 gm
Footwork	1% tolnaftate	30 gm
Rx Fungizone	3% amphotericin B	20 gm
Rx Fungoid	Triacetin	30 gm
Rx Fungoid HC	Triacetin/0.5% HC	30 gm
Rx Halotex	1% haloprogin	15,30 gm
Rx Loprox	1% ciclopirox	15,30,90 gm
Rx Lotrimin	1% clotrimazole	15,30,45,90 gm
Rx Lotrisone	1% clotrimazole/ betamethasone dipropionate	15,45 gm
Micatin	2% miconazole (T pedis)	15,30 gm
	2% miconazole (T cruris)	15 gm
Rx Monistat-Derm	2% miconazole	15,30,90 gm
Rx Mycelex	1% clotrimazole	15,30,90 gm
Rx Mycolog II	Nystatin, triamcinolone	15,30,60,120 gm
Rx Mycostatin	Nystatin	15,30 gm
Rx Mytrex	Nystatin, triamcinolone	15,30,60 gm
Rx Naftin	Naftifine	15,30 gm
Rx Nilstat	Nystatin	15,240 gm
Rx Nizoral	2% ketoconazole	15,30,60 gm
Rx NP-27	1% tolnaftate	15,30 gm
Rx Nystex	Nystatin	15,30 gm
Rx Oxistat	1% oxiconazole	15,30 gm
Rx Pedi-Cort-V	3% Iodo/1% HC	20 gm
Rx Racet	3% Iodo/0.5%HC	15,30 gm
Rx Spectazole	1% econazole	15,30,85 gm
Tinactin	1% tolnaftate (T pedis)	15,30 gm
	1% tolnaftate (T cruris)	15 gm
Ting	Undecylenic acid	27,54 gm
Rx UAD cream	3% Iodo/1% HC	15 gm
Vioform	3% Iodo	30 gm
Rx Vioform-HC	3% Iodo/1% HC	20 gm
Rx Vioform-HC mild	3% Iodo/0.5% HC	15,30 gm
Rx Vytone	Iodoquinol/1% HC	30 gm
	Iodoquinol/0.5% HC	30 gm

Iodo = iodochlorhydroxyquin

Brand Name	Generic	Size
Caldesene	Undecylenic acid	37 gm
Desenex	Undecylenic acid	27,54,480 gm
Fungacetin	Triacetin	30 gm
Rx Fungizone	3% amphotericin B	20 gm
Rx Mycolog II	Nystatin, triamcinolone	15,30,60,120 gm
Rx Mycostatin	Nystatin	15,30 gm
Rx Mytrex	Nystatin, triamcinolone	15,30,60 gm
Rx Nilstat	Nystatin	15 gm
Rx Nystex	Nystatin	15 gm
Prophyllin	Sodium propionate	30 gm
Undelenic	Undecylenic acid	30,480 gm
Vioform	3% Iodo	30 gm
Rx Vioform-HC	3% Iodo/1% HC	20 gm
Rx Vioform-HC mild	3% Iodo/0.5% HC	30 gm
Whitfield's ointment	6% salicyclic acid, 12% benzoic acid	30,480 gm
Whitfield's ointment 1/2 strength	3% salicylic acid, 6% benzoic acid	30,480 gm

HC = hydrocortisone
T = Tinea

Brand Name	Generic
LOTIONS:	
Blis-To-Sol	Undecylenic acid/salicylic acid
Desenex	Undecylenic acid
Rx Exsel	2.5% selenium sulfide
Rx Fungizone	3% amphotericin B
Rx Loprox	1% ciclopirox
Rx Lotrimin	1% clotrimazole
Micatin	2% miconazole (T Pedis)
Rx Monistat-Derm	2% miconazole
Rx Selsun	2.5% selenium sulfide
Rx Tinver	25% sodium thiosulfate
Rx Vioform-HC	3% iodochlorhydroxyquin/1% HC
SOLUTIONS:	
Rx Castaderm	Castellani paint
Desenex	Undecylenic acid
Rx Exelderm	1% sulconazole
Footwork	1% tolnaftate
Rx Fungoid	Triacetin
Rx Gentian violet	1%, 2% gentian violet
Rx Halotex	1% haloprogin
Rx Lotrimin	1% clotrimazole
Rx Mycelex	1% clotrimazole
Rx Neo-Castaderm	Castellani paint (colorless)
NP-27	1% tolnaftate
Tinactin	1% tolnaftate
POWDERS:	
Aftate	1% tolnaftate (T pedis)
	1% tolnaftate (T cruris)
Blis-To-Sol	Benzoic acid
Caldesene	Undecylenic acid
Cruex	Undecylenic acid
Desenex	Undecylenic acid
Footwork	1% tolnaftate
Micatin	2% miconazole (T Pedis)
Rx Mycostatin	Nystatin
NP-27	1% tolnaftate
Rx Pedi-Dri	Undecylenic acid, menthol, aluminum chlorhydroxide, formaldehyde
Pedi-Pro	Undecylenic acid, menthol, aluminum chlorhydroxide, starch, chloroxylenol
Prophyllin	Sodium propionate
Quinsana Plus	Undecylenic acid
Tinactin	1% tolnaftate
Ting	Undecylenic acid
ZeaSORB AF	1% tolnaftate

Size	Dose (bid-tid unless otherwise noted)
30,60 ml	
45 ml	
120 ml	10 min qd (×7d)
30 ml	4–6 times qd
30 ml	
30 ml	
105 ml	
30,60 ml	
120 ml	10 min qd (×7d)
120 ml	
15 ml	
30,120,480 ml	
45 ml	
30 ml	qd
10 ml	
15 ml	
30 ml	
10,30 ml	
10,30 ml	
10,30 ml	
30,120,480 ml	
15 ml	
10 ml	
67 gm	
45 gm	
60 gm	
60,120 gm	
45 gm	
45,90,480 gm	
25 gm	
45 gm	
15 gm	
45 gm	
60 gm	
60 gm	
2.57,120 gm	
90 gm	
45,90 gm	
75 gm	
75 gm	

appl = applicator
T = Tinea

Brand Name	Type	Generic
VAGINAL PRODUCTS:		
Rx AVC	Cream	Sulfanilamide
Betadine	Gel	Povidone
Betadine	Suppositories	Povidone
Rx Femstat	Cream	2% butoconazole nitrate
Rx Femstat prefill	Cream	2% butoconazole nitrate
Rx Gyne-Lotrimin	Cream	1% clotrimazole
	Tablets	Clotrimazole 100 mg
	Tablets	Clotrimazole 500 mg
Rx Monistat 3	Suppositories	Miconazole 200 mg
Rx Monistat 7	Suppositories	Miconazole 100 mg
Rx Monistat 7	Cream	2% miconazole
Rx Mycelex G	Cream	1% clotrimazole
Rx Mycelex G	Tablets	Clotrimazole 100 mg
	Tablets	Clotrimazole 500 mg
Rx Mycostatin	Tablets	Nystatin
Rx Nilstat	Tablets	Nystatin
Rx Sultrin	Cream	Triple sulfa
	Tablets	Triple sulfa
Rx Terazol 3	Suppositories	Terconazole 80 mg
Rx Terazol 7	Cream	0.4% Terconazole
Rx Trysul	Cream	Triple sulfa
Rx Vagitrol	Cream	Sulfanilamide
	Suppositories	Sulfanilamide
SPRAY:		
Aftate	Liquid	1% tolnaftate (T pedis)
	Powder	1% tolnaftate (T pedis, T cruris)
Breezee mist	Powder	Undecylenic acid, menthol, aluminum chlorhydroxide
Cruex	Powder	Undecylenic acid
Desenex	Powder	Undecylenic acid
Desenex for shoes	Powder	Undecylenic acid
Footwork	Powder	1% tolnaftate
Micatin	Powder	2% miconazole (T pedis)
	Powder	2% miconazole (T cruris)
NP-27	Powder	1% tolnaftate
Tinactin	Liquid	1% tolnaftate
	Powder	1% tolnaftate (T pedis)
	Powder	1% tolnaftate (T cruris)
Ting	Powder	Undecylenic acid
OTHER:		
Aftate	Gel	1% tolnaftate (T pedis, T cruris)
Derma Cas	Gel	3% phenol, 10% resorcinol
Desenex	Foam	Undecylenic acid
Desenex	Soap	Undecylenic acid
Rx Fungoid	Tincture	Triacetin
Thymol	Tincture	2–4% thymol in absolute alcohol or chloroform
Undelenic	Tincture	Undecylenic acid

Size	Dose (bid-tid unless otherwise noted)
120 gm	1 appl qd-bid (×30d)
18,90 gm	1 appl qd (×7d)
#7	qd (×7d)
28 gm	1 appl qd (×3d)
3 filled applicators	1 appl qd (×3d)
45 gm	1 appl qd (×7–14d)
#6,7	1 qd (×7d) or 2 qd(×3d)
#1	one time only
#3	qd (×3d)
#7	qd (×7d)
45 gm	1 appl qd (×7d)
45,90 gm	1 appl qd (×7–14d)
#7	1 qd (×7d)
#1	one time only
#15,30	qd (×14d)
#15,30	qd (×14d)
78 gm	1 appl bid (×4–6d)
#20	1 bid (×10d)
#3	qd (×3d)
45 gm	1 appl qd (×7d)
78 gm	1 appl bid (×4–6d)
120 gm	1 appl qd-bid (×30d)
#16	qd-bid (×30d)
120 gm	
105 gm	
120 gm	
54,105,165 gm	
81,165 gm	
81 gm	
100 gm	
90 gm	
90 gm	
105 gm	
120 ml	
100,150 gm	
100 gm	
81 gm	
15 gm	
30 gm	
45 gm	
97.5 gm	
30,480 ml	
30,480 ml	
30,480 ml	

ANTIHISTAMINES AND DECONGESTANTS

(1) *Piperazines:* Drugs of choice for urticaria, pruritus, dermatographism.
(2) *Ethanolamines:* Drugs of choice for anaphylaxis.
(3) *Ethylenediamines:* Increased incidence of GI side effects.
(4) *Cyproheptadine and Azatadine:* Antihistamine and seratonin effects.

Class	Brand Name
Alkylamines	Chlor-Trimeton, Teldrin
	Chlor-Trimeton Repetabs
	Teldrin
	Rx Polaramine
	Rx Polaramine Repetabs
	Dimetane
	—
	Actidil*
Ethanolamines	** Benadryl
	Rx Clistin
	Doxylamine
	Rx Tavist*
Ethylenediamines	Rx PBZ*
	Rx PBZ SR
	Rx Pyrilamine
Phenothiazines	Rx Phenergan*
	Rx Temaril
	Rx Tacaryl
Piperidines	Rx Hispril
	Nolahist*
	Rx Optimine*
	Rx Periactin*
Piperazines	Rx Atarax
	Rx Vistaril
Other	Rx Hismanal*+
	Rx Seldane*
Decongestants	Rx Novafed
	Sudafed
	Propagest
H₂ Blockers	Rx Axid
	Rx Pepcid
	Rx Tagamet
	Rx Zantac (150 mg*)

*Denotes uncolored preparation
**Diphenhydramine preparations may be Rx or OTC
+ Astemizole requires a median of 2 days to achieve symptom alleviation

(5) *Most sedating:* Diphenhydramine, doxylamine, promethazine.
(6) *Moderately sedating:* Azatadine, carbinoxamine, clemastine, trimeprazine, tripelennamine.
(7) *Less sedating:* Alkylamines, cyproheptadine, diphenylpyraline, methdilazine, pyrilamine.
(8) *Least sedating:* Astemizole, phenindamine, terfenadine.

Generic Name	Preparation	Dose
Chlorpheniramine	4 mg	q4–6h
	8,12 mg	q8–12h
	12 mg	q8–12h
Dexchlorpheniramine	2 mg	q4–6h
	4,6 mg	q8–10h
Brompheniramine	4 mg	q4–6h
	8 mg	q8–12h
	12 mg	q12h
Dexbrompheniramine (in combination meds)		
Triprolidine	2.5 mg	q4–6h
Diphenhydramine	25,50 mg	1–2 q6–8h
Carbinoxamine	4 mg	1–2 q6–8h
Doxylamine	25 mg	1–2 q4–6h
Clemastine	1.64,2.68 mg	q8–12h
Tripelennamine	25,50 mg	q4–6h to 600 mg/d
Tripelennamine	100 mg	q8–12h
Pyrilamine	25 mg	1–2 q8h
Promethazine	25 mg	.25–1 q8h
Trimeprazine	2.5 mg	q6h
	5 mg	q12h
Methdilazine	8 mg	q6–12h
Diphenylpyraline	5 mg	q12h
Phenindamine	25 mg	q4–6h
Azatadine	1 mg	1–2 q12h
Cyproheptadine	4 mg	tid up to 20 mg/d
Hydroxyzine HCl	10,25,50,100 mg	qid
Hydroxyzine pamoate	25,50,100 mg	qid
Astemizole	10 mg	qd
Terfenadine	60 mg	q12h
Pseudoephedrine	120 mg	bid
	30,60 mg	60 q4–6h
Phenylpropanolamine	25 mg	q4h
Nizatidine	150,300 mg	150–300 mg/d (qd-bid)
Famotidine	20,40 mg; 40 mg/5 ml	20–40/d (qd-bid)
Cimetidine	200,300,400,800 mg; 300 mg/5 ml	400–1600/d (qd-qid)
Ranitidine	150,300 mg; 15 mg/ml	300/d (qd-bid)

PSE = pseudoephedrine   PHE = phenylephrine
     PHP = phenylpropanolamine

Product	Dose
Actifed capsules	q4–6h
Actifed 12 capsules	q12h
Benadryl decongestant	q4–6h
Rx Brexin LA	q12h
Rx Bromfed tablets	q4h
Rx Bromfed capsules	q12h
Rx Comhist tablets	q8h
Rx Comhist LA capsules	q8–12h
Contac capsules	q12h
Rx Deconamine tablets	q6–8h
Rx Deconamine SR capsules	q12h
Demazin tablets	2q8h
Dimetapp extentabs	q12h
Disophrol	q4–6h
Disophrol Chronotabs	q12h
Drixoral tablets	q12h
Rx Drize capsules	q12h
Fedahist tablets	q6h
Rx Fedahist capsules	q12h
Fedrazil tablets	q8h
Rx Histaspan plus capsules	q12h
Isoclor capsules	q12h
Kronofed-A capsules	q12h
Kronofed-A Jr capsules	1–2q12h
Rx Naldecon tablets	q8h
Rx Nolamine	q8–12h
Rx Novafed A capsules	q12h
Rx Ornade spansules	q12h
Rx Phenergan D tablets	q4–6h
Rx Rondec tablets	q6h
Rx Rondec TR tablets	q12h
Rx Rynatan tablets	q12h
Rx Tavist-D tablets	q12h
Triaminic tablets	q6h
Triaminic-12 tablets	q12h
Rx Trinalin tablets	q12h

Antihistamine (mg)	Decongestant (mg)		
	PSE	PHE	PHP
Triprolidine 2.5	60		
Triprolidine 5.0	120		
Diphenydramine 25.0	60		
Chlorpheniramine 8.0	120		
Brompheniramine 4.0	60		
Brompheniramine 12.0	120		
Chlorpheniramine 2.0/ phentoloxamine 25.0		10	
Chlorpheniramine 4.0/ phentoloxamine 50.0		20	
Chlorpheniramine 8.0			75
Chlorpheniramine 4.0	60		
Chorpheniramine 8.0	120		
Chlorpheniramine 4.0			25
Brompheniramine 12.0			75
Dexbrompheniramine 2.0	60		
Dexbrompheniramine 6.0	120		
Dexbrompheniramine 6.0	120		
Chlorpheniramine 12.0			75
Chlorpheniramine 4.0	60		
Chlorpheniramine 10.0	65		
Chlorcyclizine 25.0	30		
Chlorpheniramine 8.0		20	
Chlorpheniramine 8.0	120		
Chlorpheniramine 8.0	120		
Chlorpheniramine 4.0	60		
Chlorpheniramine 5.0/ phentoloxamine 15.0		10	40
Chlorpheniramine 4.0/ phenindamine 24.0			50
Chlorpheniramine 8.0	120		
Chlorpheniramine 12.0			75
Promethazine 6.25	60		
Carbinoxamine 4.0	60		
Carbinoxamine 8.0	120		
Chlorpheniramine 8.0/ pyrilamine 25.0			25
Clemastine 1.34			75
Chlorpheniramine 4.0			25
Chlorpheniramine 12.0			75
Azatadine 1.0	120		

Brand Name	Generic	Preparation
Actidil	Triprolidine	1.25 mg/5 ml
Rx Atarax	Hydroxyzine HCl	10 mg/5 ml
Benadryl	Diphenhydramine	12.5 mg/5 ml
Chlor-Trimeton	Chlorpheniramine	2 mg/5 ml
Dimetane	Brompheniramine	2 mg/5 ml
Rx PBZ	Tripelennamine	25 mg/5 ml
Rx Periactin	Cyproheptadine	2 mg/5 ml
Rx Phenergan	Promethazine	6.25 mg/5 ml
		25 mg/5 ml
Rx Polaramine	Dexbrompheniramine	2 mg/5 ml
Rx Tacaryl	Methdilazine	4 mg/5 ml
Rx Tavist	Clemastine	0.5 mg/ml
Rx Temaril	Trimeprazine	2.5 mg/5 ml
Rx Vistaril	Hydroxyzine pamoate	25 mg/5 ml

ANTIHISTAMINES, TOPICAL

(See also: Anesthetics, Topical; Antipruritics)

NOTE: All of these products are potential sensitizers and are not
widely used by dermatologists. However, it is necessary to be
aware of these products since patients may be using them
when seen by a physician for the first time.

Dosage: Use tid-qid   HC = Hydrocortisone

Brand Name	Anthistamine
Benadryl	2% Diphenhydramine
	2% Diphenhydramine
Caladryl	1% Diphenhydramine
	1% Diphenhydramine
Calamycin	Pyrilamine
Di-Delamine	1% Diphenhydramine/
	0.5% Tripelennamine
IVarest	Pyrilamine
	Pyrilamine
Mantadil	2% Chlorcyclizine
Surfadil	1% Diphenhydramine
Ziradryl	2% Diphenhydramine

Size	Dosage
480 ml	(< 6 yrs) 0.3–0.6 mg tid-qid
	(6–12 yrs) 1.25 mg tid-qid
480 ml	(< 6 yrs) 50 mg/d (tid-qid)
	(6–12 yrs) 50–100 mg/d (tid-qid)
120,480,3840 ml	5 mg/kg/d (qid)
120 ml	0.35 mg/kg/d (qid)
120,480 ml	(2–5 yrs) 1 mg q4–6h
	(6–12 yrs) 2 mg q4–6h
473 ml	5 mg/kg/d (q4–6h)
480 ml	(2–5 yrs) 2 mg bid-tid
	(6–12 yrs) 4 mg bid-tid
120,180,240,	(See adult dosage)
480,3840 ml	
480 ml	
480 ml	0.15 mg/kg/d (qid)
480 ml	4 mg bid-qid
120 ml	(> 6 yrs) 1–3 tsp bid
120 ml	(< 3 yrs) 3.75 mg/d (tid)
	(3–12 yrs) 7.5 mg/d (tid)
120,480 ml	(< 6 yrs) 50 mg/d (tid-qid)
	(6–12 yrs) 50–100 mg/d (tid-qid)

ANTIHISTAMINES, TOPICAL
(See also: Anesthetics, Topical; Antipruritics)

Other Ingredients:

Anesthetics
  B = Benzocaine
  CM = Cyclomethycaine

Antiseptics
  BCL = Benzalkonium chloride
  CX = Chloroxylenol

Antipruritics
  C = Camphor
  M = Menthol

Drying Agents
  CA = Calamine
  ZO = Zinc oxide

Other Ingredients	Preparation	Size
	Cream	15,30 gm
	Spray	60 ml
C, CA	Cream	45 gm
C, CA	Lotion	180 ml
B, 10% CA, CX, 10% ZO	Lotion	120 ml
0.12% BCL, 1% M	Gel	37.5 gm
	Spray	120 ml
1% B, 14% CA	Cream	37.5 gm
1% B, 14% CA	Lotion	120 ml
0.5% HC	Cream	15 gm
2% Benzyl alcohol	Lotion	75 ml
2% ZO	Lotion	180 ml

(1) *Lindane:* First choice for adults for scabies. Malathion and pyrethrin are more effective for lice. 60–120 ml for whole body application. Up to 10% absorption: *Not* for children or pregnancy. Apply from chin and posterior hairline to soles of feet for scabies.

(2) *Crotamiton:* First choice for children for scabies. Less effective than Lindane.

(3) *Precipitated sulfur:* First choice for infants or pregnancy for scabies. Approximately as effective as lindane.

*S = scabies   L = lice   O = Other parasitic conditions

Brand Name	Generic	Use*
A-200 Pyrinate	Pyrethrin	L
Barc	Pyrethrin	L
Benzyl Benzoate	Benzyl benzoate	S
Rx Eurax	Crotamiton	S
		S
Rx Flagyl (also: Metizol, Metric 21, Metryl, Protostat)	Metronidazole	O
Rx Kwell	Lindane	S,L
		S,L
		L
Li-Ban		L
Rx Mintezol	Thiobendazole	S
Nix	Permethrin	L
Ovide	Malathion	L
Precipitated sulfur	Precip. sulfur	S
Pronto	Pyrethrin	L
R & C	Pyrethrin	L
RID	Pyrethrin	L
Rx Scabene	Lindane	S,L
		L
Tisit	Pyrethrin	L

Preparation	Size	Dose
Lotion shampoo	60,120 ml	Apply × 10 min
Gel shampoo	30 gm	
Liquid	60 ml	Apply × 10 min
20–25% solution		Apply qd × 2–3d
10% cream	60 gm	Apply qd × 2–4d
10% lotion	60,480 ml	Apply qd × 2–4d
	250,500 mg	250–750 mg tid or single 2 gm dose for trichomonas
1% cream	60 gm	Apply 8° qwk × 2
1% lotion	60,480 ml	Apply 8° qwk × 2
1% shampoo	60,480 ml	Shampoo 5 min qd × 2
Clothes spray	150 ml	
Tablets	500 mg	22 mg/kg bid × 5d
Suspension	120 ml	Apply bid × 5–10d
1% cream rinse	60,480 ml	Apply × 10 min
Lotion	60 ml	Apply × 8–12 hr
5–10% ointment		Apply qd × 3
Shampoo	60,120 ml	Apply × 10 min
Clothes spray	150 ml	
Shampoo	60,120 ml	Apply × 10 min
Clothes spray	150,300 ml	
Lotion	60,120,240 ml	Apply × 10 min
Clothes spray	150 ml	
1% lotion	60,480 ml	Apply 8° qwk × 2
1% shampoo	60,480 ml	Shampoo 5 min qd × 2
lotion	60,120 ml	Apply × 10 min
Gel	28 gm	
Shampoo	118 ml	
Clothes spray	150 ml	

Brand Name	Generic	Preparation	Size	Dose
Acu-Sol	Glutaraldehyde	2% soln	960, 3840 ml	3×/wk
Cidex, Cidex-7	Glutaraldehyde	2% soln	960, 3840 ml	3×/wk
Rx Drysol	Aluminum chloride hexahydrate	20% soln	37.5 ml	q3d
Formadon	Formaldehyde	10% soln	45,120, 1920, 3840 ml	qd
Rx Formaray	Formaldehyde	20% soln	45, 120 ml	2×/wk
Glutaraldehyde	Glutaraldehyde	10% soln (25%)	480 ml	2×/wk
Rx Lazer-Formalyde	Formaldehyde	10% soln	90 ml	qd
Rx Xerac AC	Aluminum chloride hexahydrate	6.25% soln	35,60 ml	qhs

Note: (1) 10% glutaraldehyde solution has been used for hyperhidrosis of the feet. Brown discoloration may occur transiently.

(2) 2% glutaraldehyde solution has been used for hyperhidrosis of the palms but is only mildly effective.

(3) 5–30% formaldehyde has been used for hyperhidrosis of palms or soles.

(4) Methenamine (5% stick, 10% solution) has been used for moderate hyperhidrosis of palms or soles.

(5) Scopolamine HBr (0.025%) topically has been used on axillary hyperhidrosis.

(See also: Anesthetics, Topical;)
Antihistamines, Topical) (Apply bid-qid)

Brand Name	Type	Generic	Size
Dodd's	Lotion	Phenol, glycerin, zinc oxide	Must compound
Lerner's	Lotion	Ethyl alcohol, glycerin, zinc oxide	Must compound
Panscol	Ointment Lotion	1% phenol, 3% salicylic acid	90 gm 120 ml
Panthoderm	Cream	2% dexpanthenol	30,60 gm
Sarna	Lotion	Moisturizer with phenol, menthol, camphor	225 ml
Schamberg's	Lotion	Menthol, phenol, zinc oxide	60,120, 240,480 ml
Topic	Gel	9% benzyl alcohol, ethyl alcohol, menthol, camphor	60 gm
Tucks	Cream Ointment	50% witch hazel, benzethonium Cl	40 gm 40 gm
Wibi	Lotion	Moisturizer with menthol	240,480 ml
Zemo	Ointment	Bismuth subnitrate, methyl salicylate, menthol, triclosan	33.8,75 gm Extra-strength 75 gm
	Lotion	Phenol, alcohol, methyl salicylate	225 ml

Note: (1) Camphor (1–3%), coal tar solution (3–10%), menthol (0.25–2%), phenol (0.5–1.5%), and salicylic acid (1–2%) also have antipruritic effects.

(2) Pramoxine is an effective antipruritic in some dermatoses when combined with hydrocortisone. (See: Anesthetics, Topical)

Brand Name	Generic	Preparation	Dose (mg)
Rx Papaverine	Papaverine	100 mg	100 4–6×/d
Rx Pavabid	Papaverine	150,300 mg	150 bid-tid

Papaverine has been used to control pruritus in patients with atopic dermatitis.

(See also: Shampoos; Corticosteroids, Topical;
Tar, Anthralin, and Ichthammol products)

This page lists preparations either expressly marketed as antiseborrheics or ones that do not fit under any of the above headings. These products may be oily preparations that are designed to loosen scale or alcohol-based drying preparations designed to counteract the oiliness of the seborrheic scalp. Ingredients include keratolytics (e.g., salicylic acid), coal tar, topical corticosteroids, and/or antimicrobial agents. Apply qhs or bid.

Brand name	Type
Rx Dermasmoothe F/S	Liquid
Diaparene Cradol	Liquid
Diasporal	Cream
Drest	Gel
Neutrogena T/Gel scalp	Solution
P & S	Liquid
Scadan	Lotion
Rx Sebizon	Lotion
Sebucare	Lotion
SLT	Lotion
Tarlene	Lotion

(See also: Shampoos; Corticosteroids, Topical;
Tar, Anthralin, and Ichthammol products)

Ingredients	Sizes
Fluocinolone acetonide (0.01%), peanut oil, mineral oil	118 ml
Methylbenzethonium chloride, emulsified petrolatum	90 ml
Salicylic acid (2%), sulfur (3%) in solidified alcohol base	112.5 gm
Benzalkonium chloride (0.125%), alkyl isoquinolinium bromide (0.15%), SD alcohol (14%)	105 gm
Coal tar (2%), salicylic acid (2%)	60 ml
Phenol (< 1%), liquid paraffin oil	120,240 ml
Cetrimonium bromide (1%) in lotion base	120 ml
Sodium sulfacetamide (10%) in lotion base	85 ml
Salicylic acid (1.8%), alcohol (61%)	120 ml
Coal tar (0.4%), salicylic acid (3%), lactic acid (5%), alcohol (66.66%), benzalkonium chloride	120 ml
Coal tar (2%), salicylic acid (2.5%) in lotion base	60 ml

Brand Name	Generic
Alcohols	40–70% ethanol, 70–100% isopropyl alcohol
Betadine	10% povidone solution
Derma Stat	65% ethanol (hand foam)
Hibiclens	4% chlorhexidine
Hydrogen Peroxide	3% hydrogen peroxide
Iodine	2% iodine (tincture or solution)
Mercurochrome	Merbromin solution
Merthiolate	Thimerosal (tincture or solution)
Phenol	0.5–1.5% phenol
Rx pHisoHex	3% hexachlorophene
Seba Nil	49% ethanol solution
Sween Soft Touch	Chloroxylenol
Zephiran	Benzalkonium-chloride (1:750)

*Triclocarban-containing deodorant soaps may be as effective as hexachlorophene soaps. (see also: Soaps)

Effects	How Supplied
70% ethanol wipe-70% reduction in bacteria (90% if left on skin 2 minutes). 40–60% ethanol equally effective but slower. 70% isopropyl alcohol is slightly more germicidal than 70% ethanol.	
Reduce bacteria by 85% for a short time. Good also for fungi, virus, protozoa yeast. Penetrates eschar.	15,240,480,960,3840 ml swab aid pads 100/box. Also available as 2% scrub (15,480,960,3840 ml), skin cleanser (30,120 ml), spray (90 ml), foam (180 gm)
(See Alcohols)	162 ml
Better than 7.5% povidone at first and long-acting but slightly less Gram-negative effect especially versus *Serratia* and *Pseudomonas.* Good also for fungi, yeast.	120,240,960,3840 ml. Also available as Hibistat skin cleanser (0.5% chlorhexidine) (120,240 ml)
Weak bactericidal. Good for debridement.	
Most effective agent for disinfection of skin but often irritating. Can be sensitizing. Aqueous solution used on lacerations.	15,30,120,480,3840 ml
Weak bacteriostatic.	30 ml
Weak bacteriostatic.	120,480,3840 ml
Bacteriostatic above 0.2%, bactericidal above 1%, fungicidal above 1.3%.	
Gram-positive (esp. *Staph*).* Slow onset but creates long-acting film with repeated use. Bacteriostatic.	150,480,3840 ml
(See Alcohols)	240,480 ml
Limited antimicrobial agent (some bacteria, fungus). Inactivates Herpes simplex virus (Type 1 & 2) if left in contact with skin for 1 minute.	60,480,630,960, 3840,19200 ml
Limited, slow-acting antimicrobial agent (bacteria, some fungi, protozoa). 1:1000 aqueous solution useful as an antiseptic mouthwash. 0.1% solution takes 7 minutes to decrease bacterial count 50%.	240,3840ml (solution) 3840 ml (tincture) 30,180 ml (spray)

Brand Name	Type	Generic
Rx Herplex	Solution	0.1% idoxuridine
Rx Stoxil	Solution	0.1% idoxuridine
Rx Stoxil	Ointment	0.5% idoxuridine
Rx Vira-A	Ointment	3% vidarabine
Rx Viroptic	Solution	1% trifluridine
Zostrix	Cream	0.025% capsaicin
Rx Zovirax	Capsules	Acyclovir
Rx Zovirax	Ointment	5% Acyclovir
Rx Zovirax	Infusion	Acyclovir (500 mg)

H = healing time   P = pain duration

Virus	Infection Type
Herpes Simplex	First episode genital only
	First episode: Genital or nongenital
	Recurrences (< 6/yr)
	Recurrences (6 or more/yr)
	Immunocompromised: First episode
	Immunocompromised: Recurrence
	Immunocompromised: Severe infection
	Ocular Involvement
	Herpetic Whitlow
Herpes Zoster	Immunocompromised: Mild infection
	Immunocompromised: Severe infection
	Postherpetic neuralgia

Notes: (1) Continuous oral therapy currently approved for 6 months at a time by FDA.

(2) Intermittent oral acyclovir gives best results if given within 48 hours of episode onset.

(3) IV acyclovir doses should be given slowly over 1 hour to prevent renal precipitation.

Size	Dose
15 ml	qh (day), q2h (night)
15 ml	qh (day), q2h (night)
4 gm	5×/d
3.5 gm	5×/d
7.5 ml	1 drop q2h (up to 9 drops/d)
45 gm	tid-qid
200 mg	See chart below
3.15 gm	See chart below
10 ml	See chart below

VS = viral shedding duration   IV = intravenous

Treatment	Comments
Acyclovir ointment q2°	H, P, VS less
Acyclovir 200 mg po 5×/d × 10d	H 50% less VS 90% less
Acyclovir 200 mg po 5×/d × 5d	H decreased 1.5d
Acyclovir 200 mg po tid–5×/d or 400 mg po bid	No recurrence 40–75%
Acyclovir ointment q2° or Acyclovir 200 mg po 5×/d × 10d	P, VS less H 50% less, VS 90% less
Acyclovir 400 mg po 5×/d × 15d then 400 mg po tid × 1–2 mos then 400 mg po bid	
Acyclovir 5 mg/kg q8° IV × 7d	
First choice: Idoxuridine Second choice: Vidarabine Third choice: Trifluridine	
Treat like other herpes simplex infections	
Acyclovir 800 mg po 5×/d × 5–10d	
Acyclovir 10 mg/kg q8° IV × 7d	
Capsaicin cream useful	

In topical therapy, choosing the proper base or vehicle for a given product is as important as choosing the proper product. A continuum model can be used to visualize topical bases:

More Moisturizing				Neutral	More Drying	
Oleag-inous Base	Anhydrous Absorption Base	Water-In-Oil Emulsion	Oil-In-Water Emulsion	Water Miscible Base	Gel Base	Soln Base

As you move to the left on this model, products become more moisturizing. The more moisturizing the product, the greasier it generally is and, therefore, the more unpleasant it becomes to most patients. As you move right on this model, products become more drying. The more drying the product, the more irritating it may be to the patient. In the center of the model are the products in water miscible vanishing bases that are neither significantly moisturizing nor drying. These products are very pleasant to the patient.

Topical therapy is really an expansion of the old adage; "If it's wet, dry it, and if it's dry, wet it." However, the physician is always balancing the degree of moisturizing or drying required for a given patient against the fact that the more efficaceous products are the ones that are generally most unpleasant to the patient. Therefore, in order to get the maximum clinical response, it is important to understand the entire continuum of dermatologic products and how to choose the proper product for each patient.

An *oleaginous base* contains no water and is completely hydrophobic. Prototypes are Vaseline ointment or white petrolatum. These products are extremely good moisturizers because they are occlusive but are often unpleasant to use over large areas of the body. However, for severely xerotic skin, usage can be very beneficial, especially after hydration from bathing.

An *anhydrous absorption base* also contains no water but has the capability of absorbing water. Anhydrous lanolin or Aquaphor ointment are prototypes. These products are generally translucent water-free ointments and are somewhat less greasy but also somewhat less effective moisturizers than the oleaginous bases.

In order to make a less oily base, the next step is to add water to an absorption or oleaginous base. However, in order to do this in a cosmetically pleasing manner, it is necessary to add emulsifying agents. The resulting *water-in-oil emulsion* will generally be white and opaque unlike the more translucent oleaginous or absorption bases. These products are somewhat less oily and somewhat less effective moisturizers than the preceding two types of bases. Eucerin cream and cold cream are examples. Some of these products will absorb additional water and have also been referred to as "hydrous absorption bases."

A few words regarding the definitions of ointments and creams are necessary. Ointments have traditionally been products containing more oil than water and would therefore encompass all three of the categories discussed thus far. However, the pharmaceutical industry has not tended to follow this definition and has used a better definition in practice. The industry has tended to call products that contain no water and are translucent *ointments,* and products that are opaque white emulsions of water and oil *creams.* By this definition, water-in-oil emulsions are considered creams, not ointments. The industry has been fairly consistent in using this definition. There are still some exceptions on the market, including hydrophilic "ointment" (an oil-in-water emulsion), which stem from an outdated definition in which all solid topical products were considered ointments. Pourable creams are generally referred to as *lotions* by the industry.

An even less oily product can be obtained by switching the proportions of oil and water in an emulsion. A product with oil in an external phase usually consisting of a larger volume of water is referred to as an *oil-in-water emulsion.* These products are relatively nongreasy, act as weak moisturizers, and are water removable but not water soluble. Many moisturizers on the market fall into this category. Nivea lotion is an example.

Products containing water and emollients that are water miscible can be referred to as *water miscible bases.* These products may be emulsions of small amounts of oil in water that are either mildly moisturizing or neutral white opaque vanishing creams or lotions. Some water miscible products containing non-oily emollients (such as glycerin) are clear liquids, and these have also been referred to as lotions. These products may or may not be emulsions. Polyethylene glycol-based products (such as PEG ointment) are also water miscible bases.

Humectants are ingredients added to many products that tend to hold moisture in the skin. The addition of a humectant makes a product behave as if it were further left on the continuum model (i.e., more moisturizing) than products with otherwise similar bases. Examples of humectants are glycerin, propylene glycol, polyethylene glycol, urea, and the alpha-hydroxy acids (i.e., lactic acid, glycolic acid, etc.). The alpha-hydroxy acids have the additional property that they decrease corneocyte adhesion and thus remove loosely adherent dry skin. The use of these ingredients allows the formation of effective moisturizers using the more pleasant oil-in-water, water-soluble, and even gel bases. However, some of the best humectants, such as urea and alpha-hydroxy acids, may cause stinging on the small fissures commonly found in very dry skin. It is often necessary to use the less pleasant greasier products to effectively moisturize these patients.

Gels are products that are translucent like the ointment bases but that consist of non-oily polymers (such as cellulose or carbomers), magnesium aluminum silicate or sodium alginate, and small amounts of solvents (such as water, alcohol, or acetone). These products are often slightly drying due to the evaporation of the solvent when the product is applied to the skin. However, if humectants are added to a gel base, it is possible to create products that are neutral or even mild moisturizers. Although these products may be water soluble, they differ from water-miscible bases by containing only a small amount of water (if any) relative to the amount of base used.

Solutions are mixtures of solutes and solvents (such as alcohol or acetone). Alcohol or acetone-based solutions are drying due to the evaporation of the solvent when applied to the skin. Propylene glycol based solutions are less drying due to the humectant effect of propylene glycol. Some thickened solutions have been referred to as lotions by the industry (for example, Valisone "lotion").

For completeness, several other bases should be mentioned.

Powders, such as talc, microporous cellulose, corn starch, calcium carbonate, magnesium stearate, zinc oxide, zinc stearate, bentonite, or titanium dioxide, act as drying agents by increasing evaporation. They are also useful in reducing friction. The addition of humectants allows a product to have a more moisturizing effect, whereas the addition of a powder gives a product a less moisturizing effect.

Shake lotions are suspensions of a powder or other solids usually in an oil-in-water emulsion. The resulting product has a drying effect due to the evaporation of water. However, the powder and oil film that is left on the skin may be occlusive enough to have a moisturizing effect. The net effect is often mildly drying but can be neutral or mildly moisturizing depending on the amount of oil in the suspension. Overall these products behave as if they were further right on the continuum model (i.e., less moisturizing) than other oil-in-water emulsions.

Pastes are made by adding powder to an ointment base. The addition of powder makes these products behave as if they were further right on the continuum model (i.e., less moisturizing) than other ointment bases. These products are most useful as protective agents.

W/O = water in oil   O/W = oil in water
mois = moisturizing

Base Category	Water Absorption	Contains Water	Water Removable	Water Soluble	Products
Oleaginous	No	No	No	No	Mineral oil, White petrolatum
Absorption (anhydrous)	Yes	No	No	No	Anhydrous lanolin, Aquaphor, Hydrophilic petrolatum, Polysorb
W/O Emulsion	Yes	Yes	No	No	Eucerin cream, Lanolin, Nivea mois oil
O/W Emulsion	Yes	Yes	Yes	No	Acid Mantle Creme, Aquaphilic cream*, Cetaphil cream (lipid free), Dermovan, Heb cream, Hydrophilic ointment, Lanphilic cream*, Lubriderm lotion, Nivea cream, Nutraderm cream/lotion, Pharmacreme, Solumol, Unibase, Vanicream, Velvachol
Water Soluble	Yes	Yes	Yes	Yes	Carbowax, PEG ointment

Liquid Vehicles	Ansel clear (A, PG), CAM lotion (O/W), C-Solve (A, G), E-Solve (A, PG), Pharmasolve AF (A), Vehicle/N (A, PG), Vehicle/N Mild (A)	A = alcohol PG = propylene glycol G = glycerin PEG = Polyethylene glycol

*Aquaphilic and Lanphilic creams may also be ordered with 10% or 20% urea.

Type	Effect
Coal tar*	Keratolytic, antipruritic, antimitotic
Coal tar*, mineral oil, + lanolin	Keratolytic, antipruritic, antimitotic, emollient
Colloidal Oatmeal	Soothing, antipruritic
Colloidal Oatmeal + mineral oil	Soothing, antipruritic, emollient
Colloidal sulfur	Soothing
Corn starch	Soothing, antipruritic
Cottonseed oil	Emollient
Mineral oil	Emollient
Mineral oil + lanolin	Emollient
Sesame oil	Emollient
Tar (others)	Keratolytic, antipruritic

*Coal tar is expressed in terms of percent coal tar in final product to allow a rough comparison of strength. Actual product may use coal tar solution, distillate, extract, etc., and these preparations differ somewhat in terms of their therapeutic properties.

Brand Name or Composition	Size
Coal tar solution (20%)	
Lavatar (25%)	120,480 ml
(Rx) Zetar emulsion (30%)	180 ml
Balnetar (Alpha Keri + 2.5% coal tar)	240 ml
Cutar (1.5%)	180 ml
Doak Oil (2%)	240 ml
Doak Oil Forte (10%)	120 ml
Aveeno	Powder 480,1920 gm
Oilated Aveeno	Powder 240,960 gm
Aveeno shower and bath oil	240 ml
Pedibath salts	Powder 30 gm (6/box)
2 cups corn starch (or 1 cup corn starch, 1 cup baking soda) to 4 cups water to make paste. Add to bathwater.	
RoBathol	240,480,3840 ml
Dermalab bath and body oil (with wheat germ and sunflower oils)	240,3840 ml
Domol	240 ml
Hermal bath oil (with soybean oil)	240,960 ml
Hermal shower gel (with wheat germ and soybean oils)	112.5 ml
Lubath	240,480 ml
Nutraderm	240 ml
Surfol	240 ml
Alpha Keri	120,240,480 ml
Cameo oil	240,480,960 ml
Jeri Bath	240 ml
Lobana	120,480,3840 ml
LubraSol	240,480,3840 ml
Lubrex	240 ml
Mapo	240,480 ml
Nivea bath oil (with soybean oil, aloe)	240 ml
Ultra-Derm bath oil	240 ml
Neutrogena sesame seed body oil	240 ml
Polytar (25%) (juniper/pine/coal tar mix)	240 ml

Brand Name	Generic
Rx Aristocort-Forte	Triamcinolone diacetate
Rx Aristocort-Intralesional	Triamcinolone diacetate
Rx Aristospan-Intralesional	Triamcinolone hexacetonide
Rx Cinalone-40	Triamcinolone diacetate
Rx Kenalog-10	Triamcinolone acetonide
Rx Kenalog-40	Triamcinolone acetonide
Rx Jac-3	Triamcinolone acetonide

CORTICOSTEROIDS, ORAL

1. If used for less than 1 month, no need for slow taper.

2. Common acute tapering regimens for Prednisone:
   a. 60 mg qd × 5d; 40 mg qd × 5d; 20 mg qd × 5d
      (30 20 mg pills/15d).
   b. 60 mg qd × 7d; 30 mg qd × 7d
      (63 10 mg pills/14d).
   c. 60 mg first day, then taper by 5 mg per day to zero
      (78 5 mg pills/12d).
   d. 40 mg qd × 5d; 30 mg qd × 5d; 20 mg × 5d; 10 mg × 5d
      (50 10 mg pills/20d).
   e. 40 mg first day, then taper by 5 mg per day to zero
      (36 5 mg pills/8d).

Brand Name	Generic
Rx Aristocort	Triamcinolone
Rx Celestone	Betamethasone
Rx Cortef	Cortisol
Rx Cortone	Cortisone
Rx Decadron	Dexamethasone
Rx Delta-Cortef	Prednisolone
Rx Deltasone	Prednisone
Rx Haldrone	Paramethasone
Rx Hexadrol	Dexamethasone
Rx Hydrocortone	Cortisol
Rx Kenacort	Triamcinolone
Rx Liquid Pred	Prednisone
Rx Medrol	Methylprednisolone
Rx Meticorten	Prednisone
Rx Orasone	Prednisone
Rx Prelone	Prednisolone

Preparation	Size
40 mg/ml	1,5 ml
25 mg/ml	5 ml
5 mg/ml	5 ml
40 mg/ml	5 ml
10 mg/ml	5 ml
40 mg/ml	1,5,10 ml
3 mg/ml	5 ml

Preparation	Moderate Daily Dose (mg)	Equivalent Dose (mg)
1,2,4,8 mg; 2 mg/5 ml	4–48	4
0.6 mg; 0.6 mg/5 ml	0.6–7.2	0.6
5,10,20 mg; 10 mg/5 ml	20–240	20
25 mg	25–150	25
0.25,0.5,0.75, 1.5,4,6 mg; 0.5 mg/5 ml	0.75–9	0.75
5 mg	5–60	5
2.5,5,10,20,50 mg	5–60	5
2 mg	2–24	2
0.5,0.75,1.5.4 mg; 0.5 mg/5 ml	0.75–9	0.75
10,20 mg	20–240	20
4,8 mg; 4 mg/5 ml	4–48	4
5 mg/5 ml	5–60	5
2,4,8,16,24,32 mg	4–48	4
1 mg	5–60	5
1,5,10,20,50 mg	5–60	5
15 mg/5 ml	5–60	5

CORTICOSTEROIDS, TOPICAL CREAM

(See also: Corticosteroids, Topical Hydrocortisone)

Base Types:	Humectants:
WM = water miscible	G = glycerin
O/W = oil in water	LA = lactic acid
W/O = water in oil	PG = propylene glycol
	S = sorbitol

*Denotes nonfluorinated product
+Class = corticosteroid strength (See explanation on page 83)

Class+	Brand Name	Base Type	Humectants	%
Rx 5	*Aclovate	O/W	PG	0.05
Rx 2	Alphatrex	O/W	—	0.05
Rx 2	Aristocort	O/W	PG,S	0.5
Rx 3				0.1
Rx 4				0.025
Rx 2	Aristocort A	O/W	G,LA	0.5
Rx 3				0.1
Rx 4				0.025
Rx 3	Betatrex	O/W	—	0.1
Rx 4	Cloderm	O/W	—	0.1
Rx 3	Cordran SP	WM	PG	0.05
Rx 4				0.025
Rx 2	Cyclocort	O/W	G,LA,S	0.1
Rx 6	Decadron	O/W	S	0.1
Rx 3	Delta-Tritex	NA	NA	0.1
Rx 5	*Des Owen	O/W	PG	0.05
Rx 1	Diprolene	WM	PG	0.05
Rx 1	Diprolene AF	W/O	PG,S	0.05
Rx 2	Diprosone	O/W	PG	0.05
Rx 3–4	*Elocon	W/O	PG	0.1
Rx 2	Florone	O/W	PG	0.05
Rx 2	Florone-E	O/W	PG	0.05
Rx 2	Halog	NA	PG	0.1
Rx 3				0.025
Rx 2	Halog-E	O/W	PG	0.1
Rx 2	Kenalog	O/W	PG,S	0.5
Rx 3				0.1
Rx 4				0.025
Rx 3	Kenalog H	O/W	PG	0.1
Rx 2	Lidex	WM	PG	0.05
Rx 2	Lidex E.	O/W	PG	0.05
Rx 4	*Locoid	O/W	—	0.1
Rx 2	Maxiflor	O/W	PG	0.05
Rx 2	Maxivate	O/W	—	0.05
Rx 2	Synalar-HP	O/W	PG	0.2
Rx 3	Synalar	O/W	PG	0.025
Rx 5				0.01
Rx 3	Synemol	O/W	PG	0.025
Rx 2	Teledar	NA	NA	0.05
Rx 1	Temovate	O/W	PG	0.05
Rx 2	Topicort	W/O	—	0.25
Rx 3	Topicort LP	W/O	LA	0.05
Rx 5	*Tridesilon	O/W	G	0.05
Rx 3	Uticort	O/W	PG	0.025
Rx 3	Valisone	O/W	PG	0.1
Rx 4				0.01
Rx 4	*Westcort	O/W	PG	0.2

(See also: Corticosteroids, Topical Hydrocortisone)

> *Possible Sensitizers:*   *Other:*
>   L = lanolin   OB = optimized base
>   P = parabens
>   PG = propylene glycol
>   SO = sorbic acid

Apply bid-tid
Elocon: apply qd

Generic	Possible Sensitizers	Size
Alclometasone dipropionate	PG	15,45 gm
Betamethasone dipropionate	—	15,45 gm
Triamcinolone acetonide	PG,S	15,240 gm
		15,60,240,2520 gm
		15,60,2520 gm
Triamcinolone acetonide	—	15 gm
		15,60,240 gm
		15,60 gm
Betamethasone valerate	—	15,45 gm
Clocortolone pivalate	P	15,45 gm
Flurandrenolide	PG	15,30,60,225 gm
		30,60,225 gm
Amcinonide	—	15,30,60 gm
Dexamethasone	P,SO	15,30 gm
Triamcinolone acetonide	NA	30,80 gm
Desonide	PG,SO	15,60 gm
Betamethasone dipropionate (OB)	PG	15,45 gm
Betamethasone dipropionate (OB)	PG	15,45 gm
Betamethasone dipropionate	PG	15,45 gm
Mometasone furoate	PG	15,45 gm
Diflorasone diacetate	PG,SO	15,30,60 gm
Diflorasone diacetate	PG	15,30,60 gm
Halcinonide	PG	15,30,60,240 gm
		15,60 gm
Halcinonide	PG	15,30,60 gm
Triamcinolone acetonide	PG,SO	20 gm
		15,60,80,240, 2520 gm
		15,80,240,2520 gm
Triamcinolone acetonide	PG	15,60 gm
Fluocinonide	PG	15,30,60,120 gm
Fluocinonide	PG	15,30,60,120 gm
Hydrocortisone butyrate	P	15,45,60 gm
Diflorasone diacetate	PG,SO	15,30,60 gm
Betamethasone dipropionate	—	15,45 gm
Fluocinolone acetonide	P,PG	12 gm
Fluocinolone acetonide	P,PG	15,30,60,425 gm
		15,45,60,425 gm
Fluocinolone acetonide	PG	15,30,60 gm
Betamethasone dipropionate	NA	15,45 gm
Clobetasol priopionate	PG	15,30,45 gm
Desoximetasone	L	15,60,120 gm
Desoximetasone	L	15,60 gm
Desonide	P	15,60,2400 gm
Betamethasone benzoate	PG	60 gm
Betamethasone valerate	PG	15,45,110,430 gm
		15,60 gm
Hydrocortisone valerate	PG,SO	15,45,60,120 gm

Note: All products below are class 6
      corticosteroid strength
      (See explanation on page 83)

Brand Name	% HC	Possible Sensitizers	Size
CREAMS:			
Rx Alphaderm (O/W)	1.0%/ 10% Urea	—	30,100 gm
CaldeCort	0.5%	L,P	15,30 gm
CaldeCort light	0.5%	P	15 gm
Rx Carmol HC (O/W)	1.0%/ 10% Urea	F,PG	30,120 gm
Cortaid	0.5%	P	15,30 gm
Rx Cort-Dome (O/W)	0.5%	P	30 gm
Rx	1.0%	P	30 gm
Cortef (feminine itch cream)	0.5%	P	15 gm
Cortizone-5	0.5%	NA	15,30,60 gm
Rx Dermacort	1.0%	NA	480 gm
DermiCort	0.5%	NA	30 gm
Rx Dermol HC	1.0%	NA	30 gm
Dermolate	0.5%	PG	15,30 gm
Dermtex HC (O/W)	0.5%	NA	30 gm
Gynecort	0.5%	NA	15 gm
Rx Hi-Cor 1.0 (O/W)	1.0%	PG	30,60,454 gm
Rx Hi-Cor 2.5 (O/W)	2.5%	PG	30,60 gm
Hytone (O/W)	0.5%	PG,SO	30,60 gm
Rx	1.0%	PG,SO	30,120 gm
Rx	2.5%	PG,SO	30 gm
Lanacort	0.5%	NA	15,30 gm
Rx Nutracort (O/W)	1.0%	PG,SO	30,60,120 gm
Rx Penecort (O/W)	1.0%	PG	30,60 gm
Rx	2.5%	PG	30 gm
Rx Proctocort	1.0%	NA	30 gm
Rhulicort	0.5%	NA	20 gm
Rx Synacort (O/W)	1.0%	PG	15,30,60 gm
Rx	2.5%	PG	30 gm

A = alcohol   F = fragrance   LA = Lactic acid
HC = hydrocortisone or hydrocortisone acetate
NA = not available   O/W = oil in water base
P = parabens   PG = propylene glycol
SO = sorbic acid   T = triethanolamine

Brand Name	% HC	Possible Sensitizers	Size
OINTMENTS:			
Cortaid	0.5%	P	15,30 gm
Rx Cortef Acetate	1.0%	NA	20 gm
Cortizone-5	0.5%	NA	30 gm
Rx Cortril	1.0%	P,PG	15 gm
Rx Dermol HC	1.0%	NA	30 gm
Dermolate	0.5%	—	30 gm
Rx Hi-Cor 2.5	2.5%	NA	480 gm
Rx Hytone	1.0%	—	30,120 gm
Rx	2.5%	—	30 gm
Lanacort	0.5%	NA	15 gm
Rx Penecort	2.5%	—	30 gm
LOTIONS:			
Rx Acticort-100	1.0%	NA	60 ml
Rx Cetacort	0.5,1.0%	NA	60 ml
Cortaid	0.5%	P,PG	30 ml
Rx Cort-Dome	0.5%	P	120 ml
Rx	1.0%	P	30 ml
Delacort	0.5%	NA	60,120 ml
Rx Dermacort	1.0%	NA	120 ml
DermiCort	0.5%	NA	60 ml
Rx Hytone	1.0%	PG,SO,T	120 ml
Rx	2.5%	PG,SO,T	60 ml
Rx LactiCare-HC	1.0% 5% LA	F	120 ml
	2.5% 5% LA	F	60 ml
Rx Nutracort	1.0,2.5%	P	60,120 ml
Rhulicort	0.5%	NA	60 ml
SOLUTIONS:			
Dermolate Scalp-Itch lotion (A)	0.5%	—	30 ml
Rx Penecort (A, PG)	1.0%	PG	30,60 ml
Rx Texacort (A, PG)	1.0%	PG	30 ml
SPRAYS:			
Rx Aeroseb-HC	0.5%	—	58 gm
Caldecort	0.5%	—	45 gm
Cortaid	0.5%	P	45 gm
Dermolate	0.5%	L,PG	45 gm
OTHER:			
Rx Orabase HCA	Orabase	—	5 gm

Apply bid-tid (Elocon: Apply qd)
*Denotes nonfluorinated product.
+Class = corticosteroid strength (See explanation on page 83)

Class+	Brand Name	%
Rx 5	*Aclovate	0.05
Rx 2	Alphatrex	0.05
Rx 2	Aristocort	0.5
Rx 3		0.1
Rx 2	Aristocort A	0.5
Rx 3	(with LA,PG)	0.1
Rx 3	Betatrex	0.1
Rx 3	Cordran	0.05
Rx 4		0.025
Rx 2	Cyclocort	0.1
Rx 6	Decaderm in Estergel (AB)	0.1
Rx 3	Delta-Tritex	0.1
Rx 1	Diprolene	0.05
Rx 2	Diprosone	0.05
Rx 3-4	*Elocon	0.1
Rx 2	Florone	0.05
Rx 2	Halog	0.1
Rx 2	Kenalog	0.5
Rx 3		0.1
Rx 4		0.025
Rx 2	Lidex	0.05
Rx 4	*Locoid	0.1
Rx 2	Maxiflor	0.05
Rx 2	Maxivate	0.05
Rx 6	Medrol	0.25
Rx 6		1.0
Rx 1	Psorcon	0.05
Rx 3	Synalar	0.025
Rx 1	Temovate	0.05
Rx 2	Topicort	0.25
Rx 5	*Tridesilon	0.05
Rx 3	Valisone	0.1
Rx 4	*Westcort	0.2

Note: Westcort "ointment" is really an oil-in-water emulsion cream.

(See also: Corticosteroids, Topical Hydrocortisone)

AB= absorption base	L= lanolin	LA = lactic acid
NA= not available	OB= optimized base	P parabens
PG= propylene glycol	SO= sorbic acid	

Generic	Possible Sensitizers	Size
Alclometasone dipropionate	—	15,45 gm
Betamethasone dipropionate	—	15,45 gm
Triamcinolone acetonide	—	15,240 gm
		15,60,240,2400 gm
Triamcinolone acetonide	PG	15 gm
		15,60 gm
Betamethasone valerate	—	15,45 gm
Flurandrenolide	—	15,30,60,225 gm
		30,60,225 gm
Amcinonide	PG	15,30,60 gm
Dexamethasone	L	30 gm
Triamcinolone acetonide	NA	30 gm
Betamethasone dipropionate (OB)	PG	15,45 gm
Betamethasone dipropionate	—	15,45 gm
Mometasone furoate	PG	15,45 gm
Diflorisone diacetate	L	15,30,60 gm
Halcinonide	—	15,30,60,240 gm
Triamcinolone acetonide	—	20 gm
		15,60,80,240 gm
		15,80,240 gm
Fluocinonide	PG	15,30,60,120 gm
Hydrocortisone butyrate	—	15,45 gm
Diflorasone diacetate	L	15,30,60 gm
Betamethasone dipropionate	—	15,45 gm
Methylprednisolone acetate	P	30 gm
		30 gm
Diflorasone diacetate	PG	15,30,60 gm
Fluocinolone acetonide	—	15,30,60,425 gm
Clobetasol propionate	PG	15,30,45 gm
Desoximetasone	PG	15,60 gm
Desonide	—	15,60 gm
Betamethasone valerate	L	15,45 gm
Hydrocortisone valerate	PG,SO	15,45,60 gm

(Apply bid-tid)
(Cordran tape, Nasalide, Vancenase: Apply bid)

Class+	Brand Name		%
GELS:			
Rx 2	Lidex		0.05
Rx 2	Topicort		0.05
Rx 3	Uticort		0.025
LOTIONS:			
Rx 3	Cordran		0.05
Rx 2	Cyclocort		0.1
Rx 3	Kenalog		0.1
Rx 4			0.025
Rx 3	Uticort		0.025
SOLUTIONS: Base: A = alcohol PG = propylene glycol W = water			
Note: "Lotions" listed below are really solutions.			
Rx 2	Alphatrex lotion	(A)	0.05
Rx 3	Betatrex lotion	(A)	0.1
Rx 1	Diprolene lotion	(A,PG)	0.05
Rx 2	Diprosone lotion	(A)	0.05
Rx 3-4	Elocon lotion	(A,PG)	0.1
Rx 5	Fluonid	(PG)	0.01
Rx 2	Halog	(W)	0.1
Rx 2	Lidex	(A,PG)	0.05
Rx 2	Maxivate lotion	(A)	0.05
Rx 5	Synalar	(PG)	0.01
Rx 3	Valisone lotion	(A)	0.1
OILS:			
Rx 5	Dermasmoothe/FS		0.01
SPRAYS:			
Rx 6	Aeroseb-Dex		0.01
Rx 6	Decaspray		0.04
Rx	Diprosone		
Rx	Kenalog		0.2
OTHER:			
Rx	Beconase AQ nasal spray		0.042
Rx	Cordran tape		
Rx	Kenalog in orabase		0.1
Rx	Nasalide nasal spray		0.025
Rx	Tridesilon otic solution		0.05
Rx	Vancenase AQ nasal spray		0.042

+Corticosteroid strength classes (1 = strongest, 6 = weakest). Adapted from Cornell RC, Stoughton RB. The use of topical steroids in psoriasis. Dermatol Clin 1984; 2:397-409.

(See also: Corticosteroids, Topical Hydrocortisone)

F = fragrance	NA = not available
OB = optimized base	P = parabens
PG = propylene glycol	

Generic	Possible Sensitizers	Size
Fluocinonide	PG	15,30,60,120 gm
Desoximetasone	—	15,60 gm
Betamethasone benzoate	PG	15,60 gm
Flurandrenolide	—	15,60 gm
Amcinonide	—	20,60 ml
Triamcinolone acetonide	PG	15,60 ml
	PG	60 ml
Betamethasone benzoate	P,PG	15,60 ml
Betamethasone dipropionate	—	60 ml
Betamethasone valerate	—	60 ml
Betamethasone dipropionate (OB)	PG	30,60 ml
Betamethasone dipropionate	PG	20,60 ml
Mometasone furoate	PG	30,60 ml
Fluocinolone acetonide	PG	20,60 ml
Halcinonide	—	20,60 ml
Fluocinonide	PG	20,60 ml
Betamethasone dipropionate	—	60 ml
Fluocinolone acetonide	PG	20,60 ml
Betamethasone valerate	—	20,60 ml
Fluocinolone acetonide	F	118 ml mineral, peanut oils
Dexamethasone (0.02 mg/sec)	—	58 gm
Dexamethasone (0.075 mg/sec)	—	25 gm
Betamethasone dipropionate	—	85 gm
Triamcinolone acetonide	—	23,63 gm
Beclomethasone dipropionate	NA	25 ml
Flurandrenolide	NA	60 cm^2, 200 cm^2
Triamcinolone acetonide	NA	5 gm
Flunisolide	NA	25 ml
Desonide (+2% acetic acid)	NA	10 ml
Beclomethasone dipropionate	NA	25 ml

The 6 class model in these charts is used with permission from Drug facts and comparisons. St. Louis: Facts and Comparisons, a division of the J.B. Lippencott Co., 1989.

These products either contain enzymes to remove necrotic wound debris or absorbant materials to decrease serous exudate in wet lesions. With enzymes, optimal results are obtained when applied tid-qid. Absorbant products are applied as needed to control exudate (often q12h initially).

Brand Name	Form	Ingredients
Rx Biozyme-C	Ointment	Collagenase
Debrisan	Beads	Dextranomer
	Paste	Dextranomer
Duoderm	Granules	Hydroactive granules
Rx Elase	Ointment	Fibrolysin, deoxyribonuclease
	Solution	(Same as above)
Rx Elase-Chloromycetin	Ointment	(Same as above) + chloramphenicol
Rx Panafil	Ointment	Papain
Rx Santyl	Ointment	Collagenase
Rx Travase	Ointment	Casein

Notes:

(A) Inactivated by some detergents and antiseptic agents (including benzalkonium chloride, hexachlorophene, iodine, nitrofurazone).

(B) Needs moist environment. Moisten wound before applying and cover with moist dressings.

(C) Must be refrigerated.

(D) Inactivated by Burow's solution, heavy metal ions (e.g., mercury, silver).

(E) Must be freshly prepared (< 24 hours old). Mix powder with 10–50 ml saline.

(F) Inactivated by hydrogen peroxide.

Type	Sizes	Notes
Enzyme	15 gm	A,D
Absorbant	25,60,120 gm packets (7 or 14/box)	
Absorbant	10 gm packets (6/box)	
Absorbant	4 gm packets (5/box)	
Enzyme	10,30 gm	E
Enzyme	1 ml vial	E
Enzyme	10,30 gm	E
Enzyme	30,480 gm	F
Enzyme	15,30 gm	A,D
Enzyme	14.2 gm	A,B,C

(Apply bid)

Products	Generic
Rx *Benoquin	Monobenzone
Eldopaque	Hydroquinone and sunblock
Rx Eldopaque Forte	Hydroquinone and sunblock
Eldoquin	Hydroquinone
Rx Eldoquin Forte	Hydroquinone
Esoterica Facial	Hydroquinone and sunscreen
Fortified	Hydroquinone and sunscreen
Regular	Hydroquinone
Rx *Melanex	Hydroquinone
Porcelana	Hydorquinone
	Hydroquinone and sunblock
Solaquin	Hydroquinone and sunscreen
Rx Solaquin Forte	Hydroquinone and sunscreen

*Warning: Benoquin is a potent, permanent agent.
Only for final depigmentation in extensive vitiligo.

Preparation	Size
20% ointment	37.5 gm
2% cream	15,30 gm
4% cream	15,30 gm
2% cream	15,30 gm
2% lotion	15 ml
4% cream	15,30 gm
2% cream	90 gm
2% cream	90 gm
2% cream	90 gm
3% solution	30 ml
2% cream	60,120 gm
2% cream	120 gm
2% cream	30 gm
4% cream, gel	15,30 gm

(See also: Bases; Sunscreens; Corticosteroids,
Topical Hydrocortisone)

Class	Emollients	Comedogenic Agents
A-absorption	CT-caprylic/capric triglyceride	DC-D+C Red 19
O-oleaginous	CO-castor oil	DO-decyl oleate
O/W-oil in water emulsion	CAA-cetearyl alcohol	II-isopropyl isostearate
W/O-water in oil emulsion	CA-cetyl alcohol	IM-isopropyl myristate
WM-water miscible	G-glycerin	IP-isopropyl palmitate
	GS-glyceryl stearate	IS-isocetyl stearate
Humectants	IM-isopropyl myristate	L(A)-lanolin, acetylated
		L(H)-Lanolin, hydroxylated
G-glycerin	IP-isopropyl palmitate	L4-laureth-4
GA-glycolic acid	L-lanolin and derivatives	ML-myristyl lactate
LA-lactic acid	MO-mineral oil	MM-myristyl myristate
PCA-sodium PCA	P-petrolatum	OA-oleyl alcohol
PEG-polyethylene glycols	PGS-propylene glycol stearate	OP-octyl palmitate
PG-propylene glycol	SQ-squalene	OS-octyl stearate
S-sorbitol	ST-stearic acid	PPG2-PPG-2 myristyl propionate
U-urea	STA-stearyl alcohol	SLS-sodium laurel sulfate

Product	Class	Emollients
A and D ointment	A	L,P
Acid Mantle Creme	O/W	CAA,G,M,O,P
Allercreme skin lotion*	O/W	CA,G,L,MO,P,ST
" (no lanolin)*	O/W	CA,IP,MO,ST
dry skin lotion*	O/W	CA,L,MO,P
" (no lanolin)*	O/W	CA,IP,MO,ST
Almay hand/body lotion*	O/W	G,GS,P,
mois balance lotion*	O/W	GS,MO,P,ST
mois renew cream*	O/W	CA,MO,STA
mois renew lotion*	O/W	CA,GS,MO,P,ST,STA
Alpha Keri mois rich body oil	O	L,MO
Aqua-A cream*	O/W	CA,CT,GS,MO,SQ,ST
Aquacare lotion	O/W	CA,MO,P,PGS
Aquaderm (C&M) lotion	WM	G
Aquaderm (Baker/Cummins) lotn*	O/W	CT,MO,P,SQ,ST
cream*	O/W	CT,MO,SQ,ST
Aqua Glycolic lotion	O/W	CA,GS,L,MO,
Aqua Lacten lotion	O/W	CA,MO,P,PGS
Aquamed lotion	O/W	CA,MO,P,PGS
Aquaphor ointment	A	L,MO,P
Aveeno lotion*	O/W	CA,G,IP,P
Betamide lotion	O/W	CA,MO,STA
Biotherm Energy Active cream	O/W	G,GS,L,MO,P
Oilfree Hydrating liquid	WM	G
Calgon After Bath lotion	O/W	CA,G,L
CAM lotion	O/W	CA,STA
Candermyl cream	O/W	G
Carmol 10 lotion	O/W	CA,IP,ST
Carmol 20 cream	O/W	IM,IP,ST
Chanel Skin Renewal lotion	O/W	G
Protectrice lotion	O/W	CA,GS,SQ,ST
Clarins treatment cream	O/W	CT,GS,MO
Revitalizing moisture cream	O/W	CA,GS,MO,P,ST
Clinique Advanced cream	O/W	CA,CAA,CT,GS,L,MO,P
Dramatically diff mois lotn	O/W	GS,L,MO,P
Skin Texture lotion	O/W	CA,GS,MO,STA
Very Emollient cream	O/W	CA,IM,L,MO,P,SQ,ST
Colladerm lotion	WM	G
gel	WM	G
Collastin lotion	WM	G

EMOLLIENTS (MOISTURIZERS)
(See also: Bases; Sunscreens; Corticosteroids,
Topical Hydrocortisone)

Possible Sensitizers	Other	Other
Dy-dye F-fragrance IU-imidazolidinyl urea** L-lanolin PB-parabens PG-propylene glycol Q-quaternium-15** SO-sorbic acid SS-sunscreens T-triethanolamine	A-allantoin AV-aloe Vera C-collagen D-dimethicone E-elastin HA-hyaluronic acid M-menthol MCL-methyl- benzethonium Cl MPC-menthol, phenol, camphor	Oat-colloidal oatmeal SA-salicylic acid SI-silicone SM-simethicone SPF-sun protection factor TiO$_2$-titanium dioxide VAD-vitamins A&D VE-vitamin E VO-vegetable oils

**releases formaldehyde

Note: mois = moisture, moisturizer, moisturizing

*Whole product tested as non-comedogenic.
Other products may or may not be non-comedogenic.

Humectants	Comedogenic Agents	Possible Sensitizers	Other
		F,L	VAD
G	SLS	PB	
G		L,PB,T	
S	IP	PB,T	
S		L,PB,T	
S	IP	Dy,PB,T	
G,PEG,PG		IU,PB,PG	A
PCA,PG	OP	PB,PG,T	A
PCA,PEG,PG		Dy,PB,PG	A
PCA,PG		Dy,IU,PB,PG,T	A
PEG		Dy,F,L,SS	
PEG			D,HA,M
LA,U(10%)	SLS	PB	
G		Dy	SA(0.1%)
PEG,U			D,HA,M
PEG,U			D,HA,M
GA(6%),PEG	L(A)	L,PB	
GA,LA,U(10%)	SLS	PB	
	SLS	PB	
		L	
G	IP		A,D,Oat
LA(4%),U(25%)		F	
G		F,IU,L,PB,T	C,VO
G,LA,PCA		Dy	
G	L(A),MM	F,L,PB	D
S	SLS	PB	
G,PG		F,IU,PB,PG,T	
PEG,PG,U(10%)	IP,SLS	F,PG	
PG,U(20%)	IM,IP	F,PG	
G,PEG,PG	MM	F,PG	A,D
PCA,PG,U	DO	Dy,F,PG,T	A,C,D,VE,VO
PCA,PG		F,PG,SO	VO
PCA	OA	Dy,F,T	VO
PCA,PG		F,IU,L,PB	D,VO
PG		L,PB,PG,	VO
PG	DO,L(A),L(H),MM	L,PB,PG	A,C,D,VE,VO
PEG,PG	IM,IS	IU,L,PB,PG	D,VE,VO
G		SO	A,C,E
G		SO,T	A,C,E,HA
G		SO	A,C,E

Class	Emollients	Comedogenic Agents
A-absorption	CT-caprylic/capric	DC-D+C Red 19
O-oleaginnous	triglyceride	DO-decyl oleate
O/W-oil in water	CO-castor oil	II-isopropyl isostearate
emulsion	CAA-cetearyl alcohol	IM-isopropyl myristate
W/O-water in oil	CA-cetyl alcohol	IP-isopropyl palmitate
emulsion	G-glycerin	IS-isocetyl stearate
WM-water miscible	GS-glyceryl stearate	L(A)-lanolin, acetylated
Humectants	IM-isopropyl myristate	L(H)-Lanolin, hydroxylated
G-glycerin	IP-isopropyl palmitate	L4-laureth-4
GA-glycolic acid	L-lanolin and derivatives	ML-myristyl lactate
LA-lactic acid	MO-mineral oil	MM-myristyl myristate
PCA-sodium PCA	P-petrolatum	OA-oleyl alcohol
PEG-polyethylene	PGS-propylene glycol	OP-octyl palmitate
glycols	stearate	OS-octyl stearate
PG-propylene glycol	SQ-squalene	PPG2-PPG-2 myristyl
S-sorbitol	ST-stearic acid	propionate
U-urea	STA-stearyl alcohol	SLS-sodium laurel sulfate

Product	Class	Emollients
Complex 15 lotion*	O/W	CA,G,GS,SQ,ST
face cream*	O/W	CA,G,GS,SQ,ST
Corn Husker's lotion	WM	G
Curel cream*	O/W	G,IP,P
lotion*	O/W	G,IP,P
Cuticura Dry Skin emulsion	O/W	CA,G,GS,IM,L,MO,ST
Cutemol cream	O/W	IM,L,P
Dermablend max mois cream	O/W	G,GS,L,P,SQ,ST,STA
Dermalab Facial mois lotion	O/W	CA,MO,P,ST
Lubricating lotion	O/W	CA,MO,P,ST
Dermassage lotion	O/W	L,MO,ST
Dior Base Fluide Lotion	O/W	CA,G,GS,IM,L,MO,ST,STA
Mois Day cream	O/W	G,GS,L,MO,ST,STA
DML lotion*	O/W	CA,G,GS,P,ST
Elizabeth Arden Immunage cream	O/W	CA,G,GS,L,MO,ST,SQ
Day Renewal emulsion	O/W	GS,IM,L,SQ
Epilyt lotion	WM	G
Esoterica lotion	O/W	GS,MO
Estee Lauder Oil Free Hydrogel*	WM	CO
Age Controlling cream	O/W	GS,L,M,O,P,SQ,ST
Eterna-27 cream	O/W	CA,IM,L,MO,P
lotion	O/W	CA,CAA,GS,IP,L
Eucerin cream	W/O	MO,P,L
lotion	W/O	G,IM,L,MO
Eversoft lotion	O/W	CA,CAA,G,IP,MO,P,STA
Formula-405 Facial cream	O/W	IP,L,MO,P,STA
Light mois cream	O/W	G,IM,SQ
moisture lotion*	O/W	GS,IP,L,MO,SA
Germaine Monteil:		
Acti Vita mois cream	O/W	CA,G,IM,L,MO,SA
Super-Sens mois cream	O/W	CA,G,MO,SQ,ST
Jergens lotion	O/W	CA,CAA,G,L
extra dry lotion	O/W	CAA,G,IP,MO,P,SQ,ST
Aloe & Lanolin cream	O/W	CA,GS,IM,IP,L,MO,SQ
Jeri lotion	O/W	L,MO
Keri lotion original formula*	O/W	GS,L,MO,
silky smooth*	O/W	CA,G,P
(Rx) Lachydrin*	O/W	CA,G,GS,MO
LactiCare lotion*	O/W	CA,GS,IP,MO,STA

Possible Sensitizers	Other	Other
Dy-dye	A-allantoin	Oat-colloidal oatmeal
F-fragrance	AV-aloe Vera	SA-salicylic acid
IU-imidazolidinyl urea**	C-collagen	SI-silicone
L-lanolin	D-dimethicone	SM-simethicone
PB-parabens	E-elastin	SPF-sun protection factor
PG-propylene glycol	HA-hyaluronic acid	TiO_2-titanium dioxide
Q-quaternium-15**	M-menthol	VAD-vitamins A&D
SO-sorbic acid	MCL-methyl-benzethonium Cl	VE-vitamin E
SS-sunscreens	MPC-menthol, phenol, camphor	VO-vegetable oils
T-triethanolamine		

**releases formaldehyde

Note: mois = moisture,moisturizer,moisturizing

*Whole product tested as non-comedogenic.
Other products may or may not be non-comedogenic.

Humectants	Comedogenic Agents	Possible Sensitizers	Other
G,PEG,PG	MM	PG	D
G,PEG,PG	MM	PG	D
G		F,PB	
G	IP	F,PB	D
G	IP	+/-F,PB	D
G,PEG,PG	IM	F,L,PG,T	A,VO
	IM,L(A)	L	
G,S	MM	L,PB,SS,T	SPF-15,VE
	SLS	IU,T	
	SLS	IU,T	D
PG,U		PB,PG	M,Triclosan
G,PEG,PG,U	IM	F,L,PG,T	A,C,VO
G,PEG,PG,U	L(A),ML,PPG2	Dy,F,L,PG,SO,T	C,D,VO
G			D,SI
G,PEG		F,L,PB,T	A,VE,VO
PEG,PG	IM	F,IU,L,PB,PG	D
G,LA(5%),PG		PG	
PG	IS	F,PB,PG,Q	C,D
PEG,PG		Dy,IU,PG,T	A,C,D
PEG,PG		L,PG	C,VO
PG	IM	Dy,F,L,PB,PG	VE,VO
PEG,PG,S,U	IP,L(A),OP,SLS	F,IU,L,PB,PG	A,C,D,VO
		L	
G,PEG,PG,S	IM	L,PG	
G,PG	IP	+/-F,PB,PG,Q	A,D,VO
PEG	IP,L(A)	Dy,FG,IU,L,PB,T	VE,VO
G,LA	IM	FG,IU,PB	A,VAD,VE,VO
PEG,S,LA	IP,L(A)	Dy,F,IU,L,PB,T	
G,PG	IM	Dy,F,IU,L,PB,PG,T	A,D,VE,VO
G,PG	MM,SLS	IU,PB,PG,T	A,D,VO
G,S		F,L,PB,Q	D,VO
G,S	IP	Dy,F,PB,Q	A,D,VO
	IM,IP,L(A)	F,L,PB,Q	AV,D
		L	
PEG,PG	L4	F,L,PB,PG,Q,T	
G		F,Q	D
G,LA(12%),PEG,PG	L4	PB,PG,Q	(150,360 ml)
LA(5%),PCA,PEG	IP,ML	F	

Class	Emollients	Comedogenic Agents
A-absorption	CT-caprylic/capric	DC-D+C Red 19
O-oleaginous	triglyceride	DO-decyl oleate
O/W-oil in water	CO-castor oil	II-isopropyl isostearate
emulsion	CAA-cetearyl alcohol	IM-isopropyl myristate
W/O-water in oil	CA-cetyl alcohol	IP-isopropyl palmitate
emulsion	G-glycerin	IS-isocetyl stearate
WM-water miscible	GS-glyceryl stearate	L(A)-lanolin, acetylated
	IM-isopropyl myristate	L(H)-Lanolin, hydroxylated
Humectants		
G-glycerin	IP-isopropyl palmitate	L4-laureth-4
GA-glycolic acid	L-lanolin and derivatives	ML-myristyl lactate
LA-lactic acid	MO-mineral oil	MM-myristyl myristate
PCA-sodium PCA	P-petrolatum	OA-oleyl alcohol
PEG-polyethylene	PGS-propylene glycol	OP-octyl palmitate
glycols	stearate	OS-octyl stearate
PG-propylene glycol	SQ-squalene	PPG2-PPG-2 myristyl
S-sorbitol	ST-stearic acid	propionate
U-urea	STA-stearyl alcohol	SLS-sodium laurel sulfate

Product	Class	Emollients
Lancome Anti-age Day cream	WS	G
Multiprotective Day cream	O/W	CA,G,GS,L,MO,SQ,ST,STA
La Prairie Cellular Day cream	O/W	L,MO,P
Cellular Balancing		
Complex lotion	O/W	GS,STA
Lubrex lotion*	O/W	CA,MO,P,PGS
Lubriderm cream	O/W	CA,G,GS,L,MO,P
lotion	O/W	CA,L,MO,P,ST
Max Factor Mois Rich cream	O/W	CA,GS,IP,MO,SQ
Soft Mois lotion	O/W	L,MO
Milk Plus 6 cream	O/W	CA,CO,GS,IM,MO,P
Moisturel cream*	O/W	CA,G,P
lotion*	O/W	CA,G,P
Moon Drops Mois balm	O/W	GS,L,MO,ST
Neutrogena Body lotion*	O/W	CA,GS,IM,
Body oil*	O	IM
Emulsion*	O/W	CA,CT,G,L(H),ST,STA
Hand cream*	O/W	CAA,G,ST
Moisture Face lotion*	O/W	CA,G,GS,P
SPF-15*	O/W	G,GS
Night Cream*	O/W	CA,G,GS,P
Nivea cream*	W/O	G,MO,P
lotion*	O/W	CAA,G,GS,IM,IP,L,MO
Extra Enriched lotion*	W/O	G,L,MO,P
Moisturizing oil*	W/O	L,MO
Visage Face cream*	O/W	CAA,G,GS,IM,L
Visage Face lotion*	O/W	CAA,CT,GS,IM,IP,MO,ST
Normaderm cream	O/W	GS,IP,L,MO,ST
lotion	O/W	GS,IP,L,MO,ST
Noxzema cream	O/W	ST
Liquid Cream lotion	O/W	CA,ST
Complexion lotion	O/W	CA,ST
Nutraderm cream*	O/W	CA,IP,MO,STA
lotion*	O/W	CA,MO,STA
Nutraplus cream	O/W	CAA,GS,MO
lotion	O/W	GS,IP,L,P,ST
Oil of Olay Beauty cream	O/W	CA,CO,G,MO
Beauty Fluid lotion	O/W	CA,CO,MO,STA
Orlane Day cream	O/W	CA,CT,G,GS,MO,P,STA
Super Mois cream	O/W	CT,GS,ST
Overnight Success cream	O/W	CA,G,IP,ST

Possible Sensitizers	Other	Other
Dy-dye	A-allantoin	Oat-colloidal oatmeal
F-fragrance	AV-aloe Vera	SA-salicylic acid
IU-imidazolidinyl urea**	C-collagen	SI-silicone
L-lanolin	D-dimethicone	SM-simethicone
PB-parabens	E-elastin	SPF-sun protection factor
PG-propylene glycol	HA-hyaluronic acid	TiO_2-titanium dioxide
Q-quaternium-15**	M-menthol	VAD-vitamins A&D
SO-sorbic acid	MCL-methyl-benzethonium Cl	VE-vitamin E
	MPC-menthol, phenol, camphor	
SS-sunscreens		VO-vegetable oils
T-triethanolamine		

Note: mois = moisture,moisturizer,moisturizing

**releases formaldehyde

*Whole product tested as non-comedogenic.
Other products may or may not be non-comedogenic.

Humectants	Comedogenic Agents	Possible Sensitizers	Other
G,PG		F,IU,PB,PG,SS,T	VO
G,PEG,PG		F,L,PB,PG,Q,SS,T	
PEG	L(A)	F,IU,L,T	
PEG,PG		Dy,F,IU,PB,PG,SO	D
	SLS	PB	
G,PEG		L,PB,Q	
S		L,PB,T	
	IP,MM	F,IU,PB,T	D,VO
		Dy,F,IU,L,PB	VO
PEG,PG	IM	F,PB,PG,Q	VO
G			D
G		Q	D
PCA,PG,S,U	L(A),SLS	F,L,PB,PG	AV,C,VO
PEG	IM,SLS	+/-F,IU,PB,T	
PEG	IM	+/-F	VO
G		+/-F,IU,PB,T	D
G		+/-F,PB	
G,PEG	II,OP	IU,PB,SS	SPF5,VE
G,PEG		IU,PB,T	D,SPF15
G,PEG	II,OP	IU,PB,T	D,VE,VO
G	DO	F	
G	IM,IP	F,L	SM
G,PEG,PG,S		F,L,PG	
PEG,PG		F,L,PG	
G,PG	IM	F,IU,L,PB,PG,SS	AV,SM,SPF5,VE
PG	IM,IP	F,PB,PG,SS,T	AV,SM,SPF5,VE
LA,PG	IP,L(A)	FG,L,PB,PG,T	
LA,PEG,S	IP,L(A)	FG,IU,L,PB,T	
PG		F,PG	E,MPC,VO
PG		F,PG,T	E,MPC,VO
PG		F,PB,PG	E,MPC,VO
S	IP,SLS	F,PB	D
	SLS	F,PB,T	
PG,U(10%)	ML,OP	PB,PG	
PEG,U(10%)	IP,L(A)	L,PB	
G,PG	MM	Dy,F,IU,PB,PG,SS	VO
		Dy,F,IU,PB	
G,LA,PCA,PEG		F,IU	C,D
LA,PEG,PG,U		F,PG,T	A,D
G	IP	F,PB	TiO_2

Class	Emollients	Comedogenic Agents
A-absorption	CT-caprylic/capric	DC-D+C Red 19
O-oleaginous	triglyceride	DO-decyl oleate
O/W-oil in water	CO-castor oil	Il-isopropyl isostearate
emulsion	CAA-cetearyl alcohol	IM-isopropyl myristate
W/O-water in oil	CA-cetyl alcohol	IP-isopropyl palmitate
emulsion	G-glycerin	IS-isocetyl stearate
WM-water miscible	GS-glyceryl stearate	L(A)-lanolin, acetylated
Humectants	IM-isopropyl myristate	L(H)-Lanolin, hydroxylated
G-glycerin	IP-isopropyl palmitate	L4-laureth-4
GA-glycolic acid	L-lanolin and derivatives	ML-myristyl lactate
LA-lactic acid	MO-mineral oil	MM-myristyl myristate
PCA-sodium PCA	P-petrolatum	OA-oleyl alcohol
PEG-polyethylene	PGS-propylene glycol	OP-octyl palmitate
glycols	stearate	OS-octyl stearate
PG-propylene glycol	SQ-squalene	PPG2-PPG-2 myristyl
S-sorbitol	ST-stearic acid	propionate
U-urea	STA-stearyl alcohol	SLS-sodium laurel sulfate

Product	Class	Emollients
Pacquin cream	O/W	CA,G,ST
Medicated cream	O/W	CA,G,ST
Plus cream	O/W	CA,G,L,ST
Pen Kera cream	O/W	G,MO
Physician's Formula:		
After Care lotion	O/W	CA,CT,G,GS
Oil Free lotion*	WM	CA,G,STA
Extra Rich lotion	O/W	CA,G,GS,IP,L,MO.
Pond's Cold cream	W/O	MO
Dry Skin cream	O/W	CA,G,GS,IP,MO,P,ST
Procute cream	O/W	CA,G,ST
lotion	O/W	CA,G,ST
Purpose Dry Skin cream	O/W	CA,GS,MO,P
Dual Mois lotion	O/W	CA,G,MO,STA
Raintree lotion	O/W	GS,IP,L,MO,ST
Revlon Dry Skin Relief lotion	O/W	CA,GS,IP,MO
European Complex cream	O/W	CA,GS,IM,L,MO
Rv cream	O/W	MO
lotion	O/W	CA,CAA,CO,STA
Sarna lotion*	O/W	CA,GS,IM,P,ST
Seabreeze Mois lotion	O/W	CA,G,GS,ST
Shepard's Cream	O/W	CA,G,GS,IM,ST
lotion	O/W	CA,G,GS,ST
Sofenol-5 lotion	O/W	CA,CAA,G,P
Soft Sense lotion	O/W	CA,G,IP,P
Sween Cream	O/W	G,L
TI-Creme	O/W	CA,GS
U-Lactin*	O/W	CA,MO,P,PGS
Ultima Daily mois lotion	O/W	CA,GS,L,PGS
Makeup mois lotion	O/W	GS,IM,L,MO,ST
Ultra-derm lotion	O/W	CA,G,GS,L,MO,P,PGS
Ultra Mide-25 lotion	O/W	CA,G,GS,L,MO,PGS
Vaseline Intensive Care lotion	O/W	CA,G,GS,L,MO,ST
Sensitive Skin lotion	O/W	CA,G,GS,MO,P,ST
Extra Strength lotion	O/W	CA,L,GS,MO,ST
Derm Formula lotion	O/W	CA,G,GS,L,P,ST
Wibi lotion	O/W	G,GS
Wondra lotion	O/W	CA,G,IP,L,P,ST,STA
Youth Garde Mois lotion	O/W	GS,L
ZnLin lotion	O/W	MO

Nail Emollients: Barielle cream (30 gm), Le Ponte liquid (9.4 ml)

Possible Sensitizers	Other	Other
Dy-dye	A-allantoin	Oat-colloidal oatmeal
F-fragrance	AV-aloe Vera	SA-salicylic acid
IU-imidazolidinyl urea**	C-collagen	SI-silicone
L-lanolin	D-dimethicone	SM-simethicone
PB-parabens	E-elastin	SPF-sun protection factor
PG-propylene glycol	HA-hyaluronic acid	TiO$_2$-titanium dioxide
Q-quaternium-15**	M-menthol	VAD-vitamins A&D
SO-sorbic acid	MCL-methyl-benzethonium Cl	VE-vitamin E
	MPC-menthol, phenol, camphor	VO-vegetable oils
SS-sunscreens		
T-triethanolamine		

**releases formaldehyde

Note: mois = moisture, moisturizer, moisturizing

*Whole product tested as non-comedogenic.
Other products may or may not be non-comedogenic.

Humectants	Comedogenic Agents	Possible Sensitizers	Other
G	ML	F,PB	
G		F,PB	D
G	ML	F,L,PB	
G,U	OP	T	
G,PEG		Dy,PB	A,AV,VE,VO
G,PEG	DC,IS	Dy,PB,Q	VE
G,PEG	IP,L(A)	Dy,L,PB	VO
		F	
G	IP	F,IU,PB,T	
G		F,T	SI
G		F,SO,T	M,SI
PG,LA		F,PG	VO
G	OS	PB,Q,SS	D,SPF12,VO
	IP	Dy,F,IU,L,PB	D
PG	IP	F,PB,PG,Q	C,D,VO
PG	IM	Dy,F,IU,L,PB,PG	C,D,VO
PCA		F,PB,T	
S		F,PB	A
PEG	IM	F	MPC
G	PPG2	F,IU,PB,T	AV, TiO$_2$
G,PG,U	IM	+/-F,PB,PG	
G,PG		+/-F,PB,PG,T	SM,VO
G,PEG		SO	A,C,D,VO
G	IP	F,PB	D,TiO$_2$,VE
G	SLS	F,L,Q	MCL,VAD
PG	DO,MM,OS	PB,PG,T	D,HA,VO
U(10%),LA	SLS	PB	
PG		F,L,PB,PG,Q	D,VO
PG	IM	F,L,PB,PG,SS	
G,PEG,PG		F,L,PG	
G,U(25%),PEG,PG	L(H)	F,L,PG	
G	L(A)	Dy,F,L,PB,T	D
PEG	L(A)	F,L,PB,T	Zinc oxide
PEG	L(A)	F,L,PB,T	
G,PEG	L(A)	L,PB,T	D
G,PEG		T	M
G,PEG	IP	+/-,IU,L,PB	D,TiO$_2$
PG		F,IU,L,PB,PG,SS,T	AV,SPF4
		PB	Zinc oxide

EPA = Eicosapentaenoic acid
DPA = Docosahexaenoic acid
Other = Other omega-3 fatty acids

Brand Name	Capsule Size	EPA mg	DPA mg	Other	# Per Bottle	Dose tid
Mar EPA Softgels	1200 mg	216 mg	144 mg	—	60	1–2
Max-EPA	1000 mg	360 mg	240 mg	—	Varies	1–2
Promega	1000 mg	280 mg	120 mg	100 mg	30,60	1–2
Promega Pearls	600 mg	168 mg	72 mg	60 mg	60,90	1–2
Proto-Chol Gelcaps	1000 mg	180 mg	120 mg	—	60,90	1–2
Proto-Chol Mini-caps	500 mg	90 mg	60 mg	—	75	2–4

HAIR GROWTH PRODUCTS, HAIR REMOVAL PRODUCTS

(A) Hair Growth Products

Rx (1) Rogaine Minoxidil 2% solution 60 ml
      Apply 1 ml bid

(B) Hair Removal Products (Depilatories)

  (1) Sulfides: Effective but bad odor, irritating
     (a) Magic shaving powder
     (b) Royal Crown shaving powder

  (2) Thioglycollates:
     Slower acting but less odor, less irritating
     (a) Better Off
     (b) Lee Bikini Bare
     (c) Nair
     (d) Neet
     (e) Nudit
     (f) Shimmy Shins
     (g) Sleek
     (h) Surgicream

(See also: Acne Treatment, Effects of Oral Contraceptives)

Brand Name	Generic	Type	Preparation	Dose
Rx Danocrine	Danazol	Androgen	50, 100, 200 mg	100–800 mg/d(bid)
Rx Nolvadex	Tamoxifen	Antiestrogen	10 mg	10–20 mg bid
Rx Winstrol	Stanozolol	Androgen	2 mg	2 mg qod-tid

KERATOLYTICS
(See also: Tar, Anthralin, and Ichthammol
Preparations; Wart Medications)

Brand Name	Components	Sizes
Calicylic creme	10% salicylic acid	60 gm
Rx Hydrisalic gel	6% salicylic acid, propylene glycol	30 gm
Rx Keralyt gel	6% salicylic acid, 60% propylene glycol	30 gm
Precipitated sulfur	3–10% precipitated sulfur ointment	
Salicylic acid	5–20% salicylic acid ointment	
Ureacin-10	10% salicylic acid lotion	240 ml
Ureacin-20	20% salicylic acid cream	75 gm
Rx Ureacin-40	40% salicylic acid cream	30 gm
Whitfield's ointment	6% salicylic acid, 12% benzoic acid ointment	30,480 gm

Apply qd-bid as tolerated.

Brand Name	Generic	Size
Rx Adalat	Nifedipine	10,20 mg
Rx Aldactone	Spironolactone	25,50,100 mg
Rx Aquasol A	Vitamin A	25000,50000 IU
Rx Dilantin	Phenytoin	30,50,100 mg
Rx INH	Isoniazid	100,300 mg
Rx Myambutol	Ethambutol	100,400 mg
Rx Niacinamide	Niacinamide	50,100 mg 500,1000 mg
Orazinc	Zinc sulfate	110,220 mg (25,50 mg zinc)
Rx Potaba	Aminobenzoate potassium	0.5,2.0 gm (dissolve in water) 100,480 gm (powder) mix 100 gm/960 ml water
Rx Procardia	Nifedipine	10,20 mg
Rx Pyrazinamide	Pyrazinamide	500 mg
Quinamm	Quinine sulfate	260 mg
Rx Solatene	Beta carotene	30 mg
Rx Streptomycin	Streptomycin	1,5 gm vials
Rx Trecator-SC	Ethionamide	250 mg
Rx Trental	Pentoxifylline	400 mg

Dosage	Representative Dermatology Uses
10–20 mg tid	Raynaud's phenomenon
50–200 mg/d	Hirsuitism
50000 IU tid	Keratinization disorders
100–600 mg/d	Epidermolysis bullosa
300 mg/d	Tuberculosis
15–25 mg/kg/d	Tuberculosis
500–2500 mg/d	Bullous disorders
110–220 mg/d	Acne, hidradenitis suppurativa
12 gm/d (qid–6×/d)	Scleroderma
120 ml/d (qid–6×/d)	
10–20 mg tid	Raynaud's phenomenon
25 mg/kg/d (up to 2.5 gm/d)	Tuberculosis
1 qhs	Nocturnal muscle cramps
30–300 mg/d	Erythropoietic protoporphyria
1 gm IM qod-qd	Tuberculosis
0.5-1 gm/d (divided)	Tuberculosis
1 tid	Atrophie blanche

Generic	Brand Name
Aspirin	Anacin, Ascriptin, Bayer, Bufferin, Ecotrin, Empirin, Norwich, St. Joseph, others
Rx Auranofin	Ridaura
Rx Diclofenac	Voltaren
Rx Diflunisal	Dolobid
Rx Fenoprofen	Nalfon
Rx Flurbiprofen	Ansaid
Rx Gold sodium thiomalate	Myochrysine
Ibuprofen	Advil, Medipren, Nuprin, others
Rx	Motrin
Rx Indomethacin	Indocin
	Indocin SR
Rx Ketaprofen	Orudis
Rx Meclofenamate	Meclomen
Rx Mefenamic acid	Ponstel
Rx Naproxen	Naprosyn
Rx Naproxen sodium	Anaprox
	Anaprox DS
Rx Penicillamine	Cuprimine+
	Depen+
Rx Phenylbutazone	Butazolidin
Rx Piroxicam	Feldene
Rx Salsalate	Disalcid
Rx Sulindac	Clinoril
Rx Tolmetin	Tolectin, Tolectin DS

*Consult manufacturer's prescribing information and the medical literature for exact dosages in various dermatologic conditions.

+Penicillamine must be given with water on an empty stomach.

Preparation	Dose Range*
325,500 mg	325–1000 qid (650 qid common)
3 mg	6 mg/d (qd-bid)–3 mg tid
25,50,75 mg	100–200 mg/d (qid)
250,500 mg	500–1500 mg/d (bid-tid)
200,300,600 mg	800–3200 mg/d (tid-qid)
50,100 mg	200–300 mg/d (tid-qid)
25,50 mg/ml	10 mg trial dose then 25–50 mg/wk
	(later reduce to q2wk, then qmo)
200 mg	200–400 q4–6h
300,400,600,800 mg	300–800 mg tid (600 tid common)
25,50 mg	25–200 mg/d (bid-tid)
75 mg	75 mg qd-bid
25,50,75 mg	150–300 mg/d (tid-qid)
50,100 mg	200–400 mg/d (tid-qid)
250 mg	500, then 250 mg q6h
250,375,500 mg	500–1250 mg/d (bid-qid)
275 mg	550–1375 mg/d (bid-qid)
550 mg	
125,250 mg	125–750 mg/d
250 mg	125–750 mg/d
100 mg	100 mg qd–200 tid
10,20 mg	20 mg qd
500,750 mg	3000 mg/d (bid-tid)
150,200 mg	150–200 mg bid
200,400 mg	600–2000 mg/d (tid-qid)

HC = hydrocortisone   Neo = neomycin   Poly = polymyxin

Brand Name	Type	Generic Name
Rx Achromycin	Ointment	Tetracycline 1%
	Suspension	Tetracycline 1%
Rx Chloromycetin	Ointment	Chloramphenicol 1%
Rx Chloromycetin-HC	Suspension	Chloramphenicol 1%/HC 2.5%
Rx Cortisporin	Ointment	Neo/Poly/HC 1%
	Suspension	Neo/Poly/HC 1%
Rx Decadron	Ointment	Dexamethasone 0.05%
	Solution	Dexamethasone 0.1%
Rx Gantrisin	Ointment	Sulfisoxazole 4%
	Solution	Sulfisoxazole 4%
Rx Garamycin	Ointment	Gentamicin 0.1%
	Solution	Gentamicin 0.1%
Rx Ilotycin	Ointment	Erythromycin base 5%
Rx Metimyd	Ointment	Sodium sulfacetamide 10%/ prednisolone 0.5%
	Suspension	Sodium sulfacetamide 10%/ prednisolone 0.5%
Rx Neodecadron	Ointment	Neo/dexamethasone 0.05%
	Solution	Neo/dexamethasone 0.1%
Rx Neosporin	Ointment	Neo/Poly
	Solution	Neo/Poly
Rx Ophthochlor	Solution	Chloramphenicol 0.5%
Rx Ophthocort	Ointment	Chloramphenicol 1%/Poly/HC 0.5%
Rx Optimyd	Solution	Sodium sulfacetamide 10%/ prednisolone 0.5%
Rx Polysporin	Ointment	Poly/bacitracin
Rx Sodium Sulamyd	Ointment	Sodium sulfacetamide 10%
	Solution	Sodium sulfacetamide 10%
	Solution	Sodium sulfacetamide 30%
Rx Terra-Cortril	Suspension	Oxytetracycline 0.5%/HC 1.5%
Rx Terramycin	Ointment	Oxytetracycline 0.5%/Poly
Rx Tobrex	Ointment	Tobramycin 0.3%
	Solution	Tobramycin 0.3%

Preparation	Dosage
3.5 gm 1,4 ml	bid–qid q3–4h
3.5 gm 5 ml	At least q3h At least q3h
3.5 gm 7.5 ml	q3–4h bid–qid
3.5 gm 5 ml	tid–qid q2–4h
3.5 gm 15 ml	qd–tid At least tid
3.5 gm 5 ml	bid–tid q1–4h
1,3.75 gm	At least qd
3.5 gm	tid-qid
5 ml	q1–2h
3.5 gm 5 ml	qd–qid q1–6h
3.5 gm 10 ml	q3–4h q15min-qid
15 ml 3.75 gm	q15min–6x/d q3–12h
5 ml	q1–2h
3.75 gm	q3–4h
3.5 gm 5,15 ml 15 ml	5×/d At least q2h At least q2h
5 ml	tid
3.75 gm	bid–qid
3.5 gm 5 ml	q3h–bid q1–4h

HC = hydrocortisone   Neo = Neomycin   Poly = polymyxin

Brand Name	Type	Generic
Rx Americaine Otic	Drops	Benzocaine 20%
Rx Auralgan	Solution	Antipyrine/benzocaine
Rx BurOtic	Solution	Acetic acid 2%
Rx Cerumenex	Drops	Triethanolamine polypeptide oleate-condensate 10%
Rx Chloromycetin	Drops	Chloramphenicol 0.5%
Rx Coly-Mycin S Otic	Drops	Colistin sulfate/Neo/HC 1%
Rx Cortisporin	Solution Suspension	Neo/Poly/HC 1% Neo/Poly/HC 1%
Debrox	Drops	Carbamide peroxide 6.5%
Rx Domeboro Otic	Solution	Acetic acid 2%
Ear Drops by Murine	Drops	Carbamide peroxide 6.5%
Rx LazerSporin-C	Solution	Neo/Poly/HC 1%
Rx Otobiotic	Drops	Poly/HC 0.5%
Rx Pediotic	Suspension	Neo/Poly/HC 1%
Rx Pyocidin-Otic	Solution	Poly/HC 0.5%
Rx Tridesilon	Solution	Desonide 0.05%
Rx Tympagesic	Drops	Phenylephrine HCl 0.25%/antipyrine 5%/benzocaine 5%
Rx VoSol	Solution	Acetic acid 2%
Rx VoSol HC	Solution	Acetic acid 2%/HC 1%

Size	Dosage
15 ml	q1–2h
10 ml	q1–2h
60 ml	q4–6h
6,12 ml	Use for 15–30 min
15 ml	tid
5,10 ml	tid-qid
10 ml	tid-qid
10 ml	tid-qid
15,30 ml	bid up to 4d
60 ml	q2–3h
15 ml	bid up to 4d
10 ml	tid-qid
15 ml	tid-qid
7.5 ml	tid-qid
10 ml	tid-qid
10 ml	bid-qid
13 ml	q2–4h
15,30 ml	q4–6h
10 ml	q4–6h

PHOTOSENSITIZERS
(See also: Tar, Anthralin, and Ichthammol Preparations)

Brand Name	Generic	Preparation	Size	Dose
Rx Oxsoralen	Methoxsalen	1% lotion	30 ml	Apply prior to UVA up to 1×/wk
Rx Oxsoralen-Ulltra	Methoxsalen	Capsules	10 mg	See chart
Rx Trisoralen	Trioxsalen	Tablets	5 mg	2 tablets 2 hours before sun exposure

Methoxsalen: Initial Dosage

Weight (kg)	Dose (mg)
< 30	10
30–50	20
51–65	30
66–80	40
81–90	50
91–115	60
> 115	70

If there is no response, or only minimal response, after 15 treatments, the dosage of methoxsalen may be increased by 10 mg (a one-time increase in dosage). This increased dosage may be continued for the remainder of the course of treatment but should not be exceeded.

Take 1.5-2 hrs. prior to UVA, (see literature for UVA dosage), up to 3×/wk.

Products	Use	Size
Chromelin	Vitiligo stain	30 ml
Dyo Derm	Vitiligo stain	120 ml
Vitadye	Vitiligo stain	15,60 ml

*Many companies produce "quick tanning" preparations that are not listed in this book.

COVER-UP COSMETICS

Products

Covermark cream, Covermark Leg Magic leg cover

Dermablend cover creme, Dermablend leg and body cover

Erace lipstick

Esteem Totally Perfect cover-up (Phone: 212-744-4660)

Liquimat acne cover-up

Note: A number of other cover-up cosmetics are also available but have not been as widely used in a dermatologic setting as those listed.

Product	Generic
Rx Anusol-HC cream	11% zinc oxide/0.5% hydrocortisone
Calamine lotion	Zinc oxide, ferric oxide
Calcium carbonate	Calcium carbonate
Covicone	Barrier cream
Dermofilm	Barrier spray
Flexible Collodion	Collodion, 0.2% camphor, 0.3% castor oil
Fordustin powder	Corn starch
Hydropel	30% silicone ointment
Ivy Shield	Barrier cream
Kerodex 51	Barrier cream (water soluble)
Kerodex 71	Barrier cream (water repellant)
pH Stabil	Barrier cream
Rx Scarlet Red ointment	Scarlet red
Talcum powder	Talc (magnesium silicate)
ZeaSORB powder	Talc, microporous cellulose, acrylic
Zinc oxide (ZO)	Zinc oxide: 12.5% lotion
	20% ointment
	25% ointment
	25% paste

* Not usable on pregnant patients.
+Corn starch is metabolized by *Candida* and can thus aggravate this condition.
NOTE: Microporous cellulose and corn starch absorb more than zinc oxide. Talc is least absorbant.

THERE ARE A NUMBER OF PROTECTIVE PRODUCTS ON THE MARKET

1. Balmex oint   (30,60,120,480 gm) with vitamin A and D
2. Caldesene oint   (37.5 gm) with vitamin A and D
3. Comfortine oint   (45,120 gm) with vitamin A and D

4. Decubitex oint   (15,60,120,480 gm) with Sulfonated Biebrich scarlet red
5. Dermamycin oint   (30 gm) with benzocaine, pyrilamine, chloroxylenol
6. Desitin oint   (30,60,120,240,480 gm) with vitamin A and D
7. Diaparene oint   (30,60,120 gm) with methylbenzethonium Cl

Size	Usage
30 gm	Protective cream with hydrocortisone
120,240,480,3840 ml	Cooling, drying shake lotion
125,500,2500 gm	Drying, absorptive powder
30 gm	Protective cream
75,400 ml	Protective spray (nongreasy) for oil or water-based irritants
120 ml	Protective film
90,240 gm	Drying absorptive powder+
60,480 gm	Protective cream
37.5,120,480 ml	Protective spray (nongreasy) for oil or water-based irritants
120 gm	Protective cream for dry or oily work
120 gm	Protective cream
60,240 gm	Protective cream
30 gm	Stimulates reepithelialization, aids in healing*
	Drying, mildly absorptive powder
75, 240 gm	Drying, absorptive powder
30, 60 ml	Protective lotion
30 gm	Ointment: ZO, petrolatum, mineral oil.
30,480 gm	
30,60,480 gm	Paste: ZO, petrolatum, corn starch

CONTAINING ZINC OXIDE INCLUDING:

8. Osti-Derm lotn	(45 ml) with phenol, camphor, Al acetate, Mg carbonate
9. Primaderm oint	(30,60 gm) with vitamin A and D, menthol
10. Saratoga oint	(30,60 gm) with eucalyptol, boric acid
11. Taloin oint	(60 gm) with methylbenzethonium Cl, calamine, eucalyptol

Also: Medicone Derma, Medicone Dressing, Medicone Rectal
   (See: Anesthetics, Topical)

Brand Name	Generic
ANTIPSYCHOTICS:	
Rx Haldol	Haloperidol
Rx Mellaril	Thioridazine
Rx Orap	Pimozide
Rx Stelazine	Trifluoperazine
Rx Thorazine	Chlorpromazine
ANTIDEPRESSANTS:	
Rx Adapin	Doxepin
Rx Elavil	Amitryptyline
Rx Endep	Amitryptyline
Rx Sinequan	Doxepin
Rx *Tofranil	Imipramine
*Contains tartrazine.	
MINOR TRANQUILIZERS:	
Rx Ativan	Lorazepam
Rx Buspar	Buspirone
Rx Dalmane	Flurazepam
Rx Halcion	Triazolam
Rx Librium	Chlordiazepoxide
Rx Serax	Oxazepam
Rx Valium	Diazepam
Rx Valrelease	Diazepam
Rx Xanax	Alprazolam

*Note: Consult manufacturers' prescribing information and the medical literature for exact dosages in various dermatologic conditions.

Preparation	Dose Range (mg)*
0.5,1,2.5,10,20 mg	0.5 bid–2 tid (up to 30 tid)
10,15,25,50,100,150,200 mg	10 bid–200 qid
2 mg	0.5–5 bid
1,2,5,10 mg	1–20 bid
10,25,50,100,200 mg tablets	10–50 tid (up to
30,75,150,200,300 mg capsules	200 qid)
10,25,50,75,100,150 mg	50–150 qhs+
10,25,50,75,100,150 mg	50–150 qhs+
10,25,50,75,100,150 mg	50–150 qhs+
10,25,50,75,100,150 mg	50–150 qhs+
10,25,50 mg	50–200 qd (tid)
+Can give in divided doses.	
0.5,1,2 mg	2–6/d (bid-tid)
5,10 mg	15–60 mg/d (tid)
15,30 mg	15–30 qhs
0.125,0.25 mg	0.125–0.5 qhs
5,10,25 mg	5–10 tid-qid (up to 25 qid)
10,15,30 mg	10–30 tid-qid
2,5,10 mg	2–10 bid-qid
15 mg	qd
0.25,0.5,1 mg	0.25-1 bid-qid

Brand Name	Coal Tar*	Other Tars	Salicylic Acid
Aqua Glycolic			
Betadine			
Beta Tar gel	2%		4%
Rx Capitrol			
Danex			
Denorex gel	1.8%		
Denorex liquid	1.8%		
Extra strength	2.5%		
Dermalab ×5			5%
Dermalab ×5/T	1.5%		5%
DHS Tar gel	0.5%		
liquid	0.5%		
DHS zinc			
Drysum			1.5%
Duplex T	2%		
Rx Exsel			
Head & Shoulders			
Herald tar	0.4%		
Iocon gel	0.85%		
Ionil Plus			2%
Ionil T Plus	2%		2%
Ionil T	0.85%		
Metasep			
Meted			3%
Meted-2			1%
MG-217	1%		2%
MG-400			3%
Neutrogena T/Gel	2%		
Neutrogena T/Sal	2%		2%
P&S Shampoo			2%
Packer's Pine Tar		0.82%	
Pentrax	4.3%		
PhisoDan			0.5%
Polytar		1%	
Protar	1%		

Other:

C = chloroxine	LA = lactic acid
CX = chloroxylenol	M = menthol
GA = glycolic acid	P = povidone
Iodo = iodoquinol	PCMX = parachlorometaxylenol

Sulfur	Zinc Py-rithione	Selenium Sulfide	Other	Sizes
			5% GA	240,480 ml
			7.5% P	120 ml
				120 gm
			2% C	120 ml
	1%			120 ml
			1.5% M	60,120 gm
			1.5% M	120,240,360 ml
			1.5% M	120,240,360 ml
				120 ml
				120 ml
				240 ml
				120,240,480 ml
	2%			180,360 ml
2%				120 ml
				480,3840 ml
		2.5%		120 ml
	2%			51,75,120,210 ml
				240,480 ml
				105 gm
				120,240 ml
				120,240 ml
				120,240,480,960 ml
			2% PCMX	120 ml
5%				120 ml
2.3%				120 ml
2%				240,480 ml
5%				240,480 ml
				135,255 ml
				90,135,165,180 ml
			5% LA	120 ml
				180 ml
				120,240 ml
5% precip				150 ml
				180,360,3840 ml
			CX	120 ml

Brand Name	Coal Tar*	Other Tars	Salicylic Acid
Sebaquin			
Sebulex cream			2%
Sebulex liquid			2%
Sebulon			
Sebutone cream	0.5%		2%
Sebutone liquid	0.5%		2%
Rx Selsun			
Selsun blue			
extra medicated			
Sulfoam			
Tarsum	2%		5%
Tegrin gel	1%		
Tegrin liquid	1%		
Tersa-Tar	3%		
Ti Seb			2%
Ti Seb-T	0.5%		
TVC-2			
Vanseb cream			1%
Vanseb lotion			1%
Vanseb-T cream	1%		1%
Vanseb-T lotion	1%		1%
X-seb			4%
X-seb-T	2%		4%
Zetar	1%		
Zincon			
ZNP Bar			

EFFECTS OF INDIVIDUAL INGREDIENTS

	Coal Tar*	Other Tars	Salicylic Acid
Antibacterial	*	*	
Antifungal			
Antimitotic	*	*	
Antipruritic	*	*	*
Cytotoxic			
Keratolytic	*	*	*

*Coal Tar is expressed in terms of percent coal tar in final product, to allow a rough comparison of strength. Actual product may use coal tar solution, distillate, extract, etc., and these preparations differ somewhat in terms of their therapeutic properties.

Fragrance and color-free shampoos:

— DHS clear   240,480 ml
— Duplex   480,3840 ml (no sensitizers)

Other:

C = chloroxine	LA = lactic acid
CX = chloroxylenol	M = menthol
GA = glycolic acid	P = povidone
Iodo = iodoquinol	PCMX = para-chloro-metaxylenol

Sulfur	Zinc Pyrithione	Selenium Sulfide	Other	Sizes
			3% Iodo	120 ml
2%				120 gm
2%				120,240 ml
	2%			120,240 ml
2%				120 gm
2%				120,240 ml
		2.5%		120 ml
		1.0%		120,210,330 ml
		1.0%	0.5% M	120,210,330 ml
2%				120,240,465 ml
				120 ml
				75 gm
				112.5,198 ml
				240 ml
				240 ml
				240 ml
	2%			120 ml
2%				90 gm
2%				120 ml
2%				90 gm
2%				120 ml
				120 ml
				120 ml
				180 ml
	1%			120,240 ml
	2%			126 gm

Sulfur	Zinc Pyrithione	Selenium Sulfide	Other	
*	*		C, Iodo, LA, P, PCMX	
*	*	*	Iodo, P	
		*		
			M	
	*			
*			GA, LA	

(See also: Antiseptics for Betadine, Hibiclens, pHisoHex, Seba Nil)

IRRITANCY:

Relative irritancy of soaps has been a controversial subject. The Finn chamber test measures irritancy when soap is left in continuous contact with the skin for lengths of time far exceeding normal washing. The pH of the skin is mildly acidic. Basic pH soaps (such as Basis) generally have tested more irritating using the Finn chamber because prolonged application overwhelms the buffering capacity of the stratum corneum. Since soaps are not generally left in contact with the skin for prolonged periods, the Finn chamber may overestimate the irritancy of basic pH soaps.

(Best to Worst—Finn Chamber Test)

  (1) Cetaphil
  (2) Dove
  (3) Aveeno
  (4) Alpha Keri, Dial, Fels Naphtha, Irish Spring, Neutrogena, Purpose, Safeguard
  (5) Ivory, Oilatum, Lowila, Jergens, Lubriderm
  (6) Cuticura, Basis
  (7) Zest, Camay, Lava

LOW pH (< 7.5):   *ALSO:*

3.5—4.4	pHresh, Fostex, Lowila	Alpha Keri, Caress,
4.5—4.9	Aveeno (dry or acne), Buf	Dermalab skin cleanser,
5.0—5.4	Amino-Pon, Climatress	Doak Tersaseptic
5.5	Drytergent, Eucerin,	(nonsoap cleanser),
	Night Cast Skin Cleanser,	Emulave, Neutrogena,
	Sween Kind Touch,	PanOxyl 5 or 10,
	Sween Soft Touch	pHisoDerm, (RX) pHisoHex,
5.6—5.9	Acnaveen, Aveeno	Physician's Formula-
	(normal/oily), Bio-clear	gentle cleansing lotion,
6.2—7.0	Cetaphil, Dove	Purpose

NONSOAP CLEANSERS:

Alpha Keri Gelee (with collagen), Aveeno (dry, acne, normal/oily), Doak Tersaseptic, Dermalab skin cleanser, Drytergent, Duplex, Estee Lauder basic cleansing bar, Keri facial cleanser, Lowila, Moisturel sensitive skin cleanser, Night Cast skin cleanser, pHisoDerm, Physician's Formula deep cleanser, SFC lotion, Sulfoil

---

LIPID-FREE CLEANSERS:

Lipid-free cleansers are often tolerated by atopic patients who cannot tolerate even mild soaps.

      Aquanil, Beta Care cream or lotion
      CAM Lotion, Cetaphil,
(Rx) Cetacort (with 0.25, 0.5, or 1% hydrocortisone)
      Drytergent, Duplex

SUPERFATTED

Superfatted soaps attempt to act as mild moisturizers by depositing oil on the skin in excess of that removed by the soap during washing. Many of these soaps have a basic pH and have tested poorly in the Finn chamber. However, as previously mentioned, the Finn chamber may overestimate the irritancy of basic pH soaps. There is evidence that some of these soaps (such as Basis) and certain surfactant bars (such as Dove) leave the skin less rough than standard soaps. However, soaps generally test better than surfactant bars at preventing cutaneous water loss.

Alpha Keri moisturizing bar, Aveeno (dry skin), Basis, Camay, Clinique facial soap mild, Dermalab superfatted, Lubriderm, Nivea soap, Oilatum, Petro-phylic soap, Shepard's soap

---

LAUNDRY DETERGENT FOR SENSITIVE SKIN:

Safeskin

TAR SOAPS:

Polytar, Packer's Pine Tar, Tegrin

PERIANAL CLEANSERS:

Balneol lotion,
Mediconet wipes (50% witch hazel, 0.02% BCL),
Peri-Wash, Peri-Wash II,
Preparation H cleansing pads (50% witch hazel),
Rantex wipes (BCL, 50% witch hazel),
Tucks pads (50% witch hazel, 0.003% BCL)

(BCL = benzalkonium chloride)

BA = benzoic acid
BPO = benzoyl peroxide

BCL = benzalkonium chloride
S = sulfur   SA = salicylic acid

ACNE SOAPS AND CLEANSERS:

A number of soaps have been designed for use by acne patients, and many of these are listed below. The deodorant soaps, which contain antimicrobial agents triclocarban or triclosan, are also useful in acne and often represent a less expensive alternative choice.

Acne-Aid Cleansing Bar
Acno astringent/cleanser
Aqua Glyde (2.5% glycolic acid)
Aveeno cleansing bar (2% S, 2% SA)
Rx Benzac W Lotion (5, 10% BPO wash)
Brasivol cream (abrasive)
Buf bar (3% sulfur)
Buf Puff antiseptic cleanser (0.13 BCL, alcohol)
Clearasil antibacterial bar
Clearasil astringent/cleanser (SA)
Rx Desquam-X (5,10% BPO wash, 10% bar)
Dry and Clear cleanser (0.5% SA,
   0.5% BA, 0.1% Benzethonium Cl)
Drytex (SA)
Fostex 10% bar/wash (10% BPO)
Fostex medicated bar (2% S, 2% SA)
Ionax (foam/cleanser) (1.4% SA)
Ionax scrub (abrasive)
Komex scrub (abrasive)
Listerex scrub (2% SA)
Neutrogena extra mild acne cleanser
Noxzema clear-up pads (0.5% SA)
Noxzema skin cleanser-regular/extra strength (alcohol)
Noxzema skin cleanser-sensitive skin (0.13% BCL)
Oxy Clean soap (3.5% S)
Oxy Clean cleanser, pads (0.5% SA)
Oxy-scrub (abrasive)
Oxy 10 wash (10% BPO)
PanOxyl (5,10% BPO bars)
Pernox soap (abrasive, 2% S, 1.5% SA)
Pernox lotion (abrasive, 2% S, 2% SA)
Propa pH soap (10% BPO wash)
SalAc lotion (2% SA)
SAStid cleanser (1.6% S, 1.6% SA)
SAStid soap (10% S, 3% SA) (Also: SA, S, SA+S soaps)
SAStid AL scrub (abrasive, 1.6% S, 1.6% SA)
Seba-Nil cleanser
Seba-Nil cleansing mask (abrasive)
Seba-Nil liquid (alcohol)
Stridex pads, regular (0.5% SA)
Stridex pads, maximum strength (2% SA)
Sulpho-lac soap (5% S)
Tyrosum cleanser and pads (alcohol)

DEODORANT SOAPS:

Triclosan — Lifebuoy, Phase III, Clearasil Soap
Triclocarban — Coast, Cuticura, Irish Spring, Dial,
Jergens, Safeguard, Zest

Sunscreens	UV Spectrum (nm)
Benzophenones	
Oxybenzone	270–350
Dioxybenzone	260–380
PABA and PABA esters	
p-aminobenzoic acid	260–313
Padimate O (octyl dimethyl PABA)	290–315
Glyceryl PABA	264–315
Cinnamates	
Ethylhexyl-p-methoxycinnamate	290–320*
Cinoxate	270–328
Salicylates	
Octylsalicylate	280–320
Homosalate	290–315
Miscellaneous	
Methyl anthranilate	290–320*
Digalloyl trioleate	270–320
Butyl Methoxydibenzoylmethane	320–400
Titanium dioxide	290–700
Red Petrolatum	290–365**
Zinc oxide	290–700

UVC — < 290 nm
UVB — 290–320 nm
UVA — 320–400 nm
Visible light — > 400 nm

*May provide some limited UVA protection.
**Provides only partial protection in UVA portion of spectrum.

Adapted and used with permission from
Drug facts and comparisons. St. Louis:
Facts and Comparisons, a division of the J.B. Lippencott Co., 1989.

B = Benzophenones
M = Moisturizing
P = PABA
PE = PABA ester
EPC = Ethylhexyl-p-methoxycinnamate

OC = Other cinnamates
S = Salicylates
SPF = Sun protection factor
T = Titanium dioxide

Brand Name	SPF	M	P
Alo Sun Fashion Tan	4		
Fashion Tan	8		
Fashion Tan	15		
Aqua Ray Lotion	22		
Bain de Soleil Deep Tanning Creme	2		
Gelee	4		
Gelee Stick	4		
Oil	4		
Creme	6		
Gelee	10		
Creme	15	X	
Spray Lotion	15	X	
Gelee Stick	15		
Spray Lotion	20		
Creme	25		
Stick	25		
Biotherm Bronzing Gel	4		
Tanning Lotion	8	X	
Oil Free Sun Gel	10		
Sun Stick	10		
Bullfrog Gel	9		
Gel	18		
Stick	18		
Gel	36		
Chanel Bronzing Mist	4		
Bronzing Lotion	8	X	
Oil Free Bronzing Mist	10		
Sun Shelter Cream	15	X	
Oil Free Sun Shelter Lotion	23		
Clarins Sun Care Oil	2	X	
Deep Tanning Gel	4	X	
Sun Care Milk	9	X	
Sun Wrinkle Control Cream	10	X	
Total Sunscreen Emulsion	18	X	
Clinique Sun Block	19	X	
Coppertone Dark Tanning Oil	2		
Dark Tanning Spray	2		
Lite Tanning Lotion	4		
Lotion	4		
Lotion	6		
Lotion	8		
Oil Free Lotion	10		
Lotion	15		
Lotion	25		
Lotion	30+		
Lotion	44		

Other:
O = Octocrylene

PE	B	EPC	OC	S	T	Other
X						
X	X					
X	X					
	X		X	X		
X	X					
X		X				
X		X				
X		X				
X	X					
X	X	X				
X	X	X				
X	X	X				
X	X	X				
X	X	X				
	X		X			
	X		X			
	X		X	X		
	X		X			
	X		X			
X			X			O
	X		X			O
	X		X			
	X		X			
	X		X			
	X		X	X		
X	X		X	X		
	X		X			
	X		X			
	X		X			
	X		X			
	X		X			
X	X		X			
				X		
X				X		
X	X					
X	X					
X	X					
	X	X		X		
	X	X				
X						
X		X				
X	X	X		X		
X	X	X		X		

B = Benzophenones
M = Moisturizing
P = PABA
PE = PABA ester
EPC = Ethylhexyl-p-methoxycinnamate
OC = Other cinnamates
S = Salicylates
SPF = Sun protection factor
T = Titanium dioxide

Brand Name	SPF	M	P
Dermablend Maximum Moisturizer Cream	15	X	
Dermalab Sunscreen Lotion	4		
Sunscreen Lotion	8		
Sunblock Lotion	15		
Total Sun Block Lotion	23		
Eclipse Original	10		
Partial Eclipse Lotion	6		
Total Eclipse Mois Lotion	15	X	
Cooling Alcohol Lotion	15		
Lotion	20		
Lotion	25		
Solar Blok Cream	33		
Estee Lauder Golden Bronzing Oil	3	X	
Oil Free Tanning Formula Lotion	6		
Sport Bronzer Lotion	8		
Oil Free Sun Spray	10		
Waterworld Sunscreen Lotion	15		
Super Sun Block Lotion	20		
Sun Out Lotion	34		
Formula 405 Solar lotion	8		
Solar Cream	15	X	X
Germaine Monteil Soleil Creme	25	X	
Hawaiian Tropic Dark Tanning Oil	2		
Professional Light Tanning Oil	2		
Dark Tanning Lotion	4		
Dark Tanning Lotion Extra	4		
Protective Tanning Lotion	6		
Protective Tanning Dry Oil	6		
Aloe PABA Cream	8		
Swim N Sun Lotion	10		
15 Sunblock Spray	15		
15 Plus Sunblock	15		
Swim N Sun Gel	20		
Baby Faces Lotion	22		
Baby Faces Lotion	25		
Ozone Sunblock	30		
Lancaster Sun Oil	2		
Tanning Emulsion	4	X	
Tanning Emulsion	6	X	
Sensitive Sun Cream	6		
High Altitude Creme	8	X	
High Protection Cream	8		
Sun Protecting Stick	8		
Lancome Anti-Wrinkle Sun Cream	6	X	
Oil Free Sun Spray	10		
Sunblock Creme	15	X	
Waterproof Body Sun Block Lotion	15	X	
Maximum Sun Block Lotion	23	X	
Neutrogena PABA-Free Sunblock Cream	15		

Other:
MA = Methylanthranilate

PE	B	EPC	OC	S	T	Other
	X		X			
	X	X				
	X	X				
	X	X				
X	X	X				
X						
X						
X	X			X		
X	X					
X	X		X			
	X			X	X	
X	X		X		X	
	X		X			
	X		X			
			X			
	X		X	X		
	X		X	X		
	X		X	X		
X	X		X			
			X			
					X	
	X		X			
X		X				
	X	X				
	X		X			
X		X				
X	X					
X	X					
X	X					
X	X					
X	X	X				
X	X					
X	X	X				
X	X		X			
	X	X		X		MA
X	X	X				
			X			
X			X			
X			X			
X			X			
X			X			
X			X			
X	X		X			
	X		X			
	X		X			
X	X					
X	X					
X	X		X			
	X		X			

B = Benzophenones
M = Moisturizing
P = PABA
PE = PABA ester
EPC = Ethylhexyl-p-methoxycinnamate
OC = Other cinnamates
S = Salicylates
SPF = Sun protection factor
T = Titanium dioxide

Brand Name	SPF	M	P
Pabanol Lotion	14		X
Photoplex Lotion	15	X	
Piz Buin Lotion	8		
Lotion	15		
Cream	15		
Lotion	25		
Pre Sun Creamy Lotion	4		
Creamy Cream	8		
Gel	8		
Lotion	8		X
Creamy Cream	15	X	
Lotion	15		
Lotion	29		
Lotion	39		
Q T Lotion	2		
Rene Guinot UV Filtre Total Cream	7		
Sea & Ski Lotion	4		
Lotion	6		
Lotion	15		
Blockout Clear Lotion	15		
Blockout Creme Lotion	15		
Blockout Creme Lotion	30	X	
Shade Lotion	6		
Lotion	8		
Plus Lotion	8		
Supershade Lotion	8		
Supershade Lotion	15		
Supershade Oilfree Clear Gel	15		
Supershade Lotion	25		
Supershade Stick	25		
Supershade Lotion	30		
Supershade Lotion	44		
Solbar PF 15 Cream	15		
PF 15 Liquid	15		
Plus 15 Cream	15		
PF 50 Cream	50		
Sun Basics Sun Care Cream	6		
Sundown Lotion	4		
Lotion	6		
Lotion	8		
Lotion	15		
Stick	15		
Lotion	20		
Stick	20		
Creme	24		
Broad Spectrum Lotion	15		
Broad Spectrum Lotion	25		
Broad Spectrum Lotion	30		

Other:
BMD = Butyl methoxydibenzolymethane
MA = Methylanthranilate
O = Octocrylene

PE	B	EPC	OC	S	T	Other
X						BMD
	X		X			
	X		X			
	X		X		X	
	X		X	X	X	
X						
X	X					
X	X					
X	X					
X	X		X	X		
X	X					
X						
	X					
X						
X						
X	X		X			
			X	X		
X	X		X			
X	X		X			
X	X					
X	X					
X	X					
X	X					
	X	X				
	X	X				
X	X	X				
	X	X		X		
	X	X		X		MA
X	X	X		X		
X	X	X		X		
	X		X			
	X		X			
X	X					
	X		X			O
X						
X	X					
X	X					
X	X					
X	X		X			
X	X					
X	X		X		X	
X			X		X	
X	X					
	X		X	X	X	
	X		X	X	X	
	X		X	X	X	

B = Benzophenones
M = Moisturizing
P = PABA
PE = PABA ester
EPC = Ethylhexyl-p-methoxycinnamate

OC = Other cinnamates
S = Salicylates
SPF = Sun protection factor
T = Titanium dioxide

Brand Name	SPF	M	P
Sun Science (Elizabeth Arden)			
Spot-Protection Sunblock	15	X	
Oil-Free Ultra Block	15		
Lotion	34	X	
Sunsitive (Hawaiian Tropic)			
Professional Tanning Dry Oil	5		
Professional Tanning Milk	5		
Dry Lotion Sunblock	15		
15 Spray Sunblock	15		
Soft Lotion Sunblock	30		
TI-Screen Lotion	8		
Lotion	15+		
Lotion	20+		
Lotion	30+		
Tropical Blend Lotion	2		
Lotion	4		
Lotion	5		
Lotion	8		
Lotion	15		
Lotion	30		
Vaseline Intensive Care Lotion	2	X	
Lotion	4	X	
Lotion	8	X	
Lotion	15	X	
Lotion	25	X	
Water Babies (Coppertone) Lotion	15	X	
Lotion	25	X	
Lotion	30	X	
CHILDREN'S SUNSCREENS:			
Johnson's Baby Sunblock Cream	15		
Lotion	15		
Pre Sun Children's Lotion	29		
Sea & Ski Baby Lotion	2		
Blockout Spray for Kids	28		
Blockout Creme Lotion for Kids	30		
TI-Screen Baby	15+		
EYE SUNSCREENS:			
Bain de Soleil Under Eye Protector	30		
Lancaster Sun Eye Care	8		
Lancome Eye and Lip Protector	12		
Waterproof Eye and Lip Protector	12		
Sun Basics Sun Care for Lips and Eyes	15		

Other:
MA = Methylanthranilate
 O = Octocrylene

PE	B	EPC	OC	S	T	Other
X	X					
X	X					
X	X					
	X	X				MA
		X				MA
		X				MA
		X				MA
	X	X		X		MA
	X	X				
	X	X				
	X	X		X		
	X	X		X		O
				X		
X	X					
	X	X				
X	X			X		
X	X	X		X		
	X	X		X		
		X				
	X	X				
	X	X				
	X	X				
	X	X				
	X	X				
	X	X		X		
	X	X		X		
	X		X	X	X	
	X		X	X	X	
	X		X	X		
X						
X	X		X	X		
X	X	X	X			
	X	X				
	X	X		X		
X			X			
	X		X			
X	X					
X	X					

B = Benzophenones
EPC = Ethylhexyl-p-
     methoxycinnamate
M = Moisturizing
OC = Other cinnamates

P = PABA
PE = PABA ester
S = Salicylates
SPF = Sun protection
      factor
T = Titanium
    dioxide

Brand Name	SPF	M	P
FACIAL SUNSCREENS:			
Bain de Soleil Facial Creme	6		
Facial Creme	15	X	
Facial Creme	25	X	
Chanel Sun Shelter Face Block	15		
Clinique Face Zone Cream	15		
Estee Lauder Sun Stick Face	15		
Total Face Block	25		
Neutrogena Facial Sunscreen	15		
Pre Sun Stick, Face	15		
TI-Screen Lip and Face	15+		
Total Eclipse Lip & Face	15		
LIP SUNSCREENS:			
Bain de Soleil Lip Protector	30		
Blistex Daily Conditioning Lip Balm	15		
Blistik Lip Balm	10		
Chapstick Lip Balm	15		
Hawaiian Tropic Lip Balm	15		
Lancome Eye and Lip Protector	12		
Waterproof Eye and Lip Protector	12		
Lipkote	15		
Neutrogena Lip Moisturizer	15	X	
Pfeiffer Lip Treatment	15	X	
Physician's Formula Lip Care	15		
Pre Sun Lip	15		
RVPaba Lipstick	SB		X
Sun Basics Sun Care for Lips and Eyes	15		
TI-Screen Lip and Face	15+		
Total Eclipse Lip & Face	15		
Vaseline Lip Therapy	15		
NOSE SUNSCREENS:			
Alosun Nose Shield	15		
Nosekote Cream	8		
Cream	15		
Snootie (Sea & Ski)	10		
SCALP SUNSCREENS:			
Alosun Top Kote Scalp Lotion	15		
SUNBLOCKS:			
Afil Cream	SB		
Maxafil Cream	SB	X	
RVP	SB		
RVPaque	SB		
RVPaba Lipstick	SB		X
Zinka Cream	SB		

Other:
MA = Methylanthranilate
RP = Red petrolatum
SB = Sunblock
ZO = Zinc oxide

PE	B	EPC	OC	S	T	Other
X	X					
X	X					
X	X	X				
X	X					
	X		X			
	X		X			
	X		X	X		
X	X					
X	X					
	X	X				
X	X					
	X	X		X		
X	X					
X	X					
X	X					
X	X					
	X		X			
X	X					
X	X					
X	X					
X	X					
X	X					
						RP
X	X					
	X	X				
X	X					
X	X					
	X		X			
	X			X		
X	X					
X						
X	X					
					X	MA
			X			MA
						RP
		X				RP,ZO
						RP
					X	ZO

(See also: Soaps, Baths, Shampoos)

LCD = Liquid carbonis detergens   SA = salicylic acid
     = coal tar solution
     = 20% crude coal tar

Generic Preparation	Brand Name
ANTHRALIN CREAMS:	Rx Drithocreme
	Rx Drithocreme HP
	Rx Drithoscalp
	Rx Lasan cream
	Rx Lasan HP cream
ANTHRALIN OINTMENT:	Rx Anthra-Derm ointment
	Rx Lasan ointment
ANTHRALIN PASTES:	Rx Anthralin paste
COAL TAR CREAMS:	Alphosyl
	Rx Fototar
	Mazon
	Tegrin
COAL TAR OINTMENTS:	Rx Crude coal tar in petrolatum
	Medotar
	MG-217
	Taraphilic
	Rx Unguentum Bossi
COAL TAR LOTIONS, OILS, and SOLUTIONS:	Alphosyl Lotion
	Balnetar oil
	Doak tar lotion
	Neutrogena T/Derm oil
	Neutrogena T/Gel scalp solution
	Neutrogena T/Gel therapeutic conditioner (lotion)
	Oxipor-VHC Lotion
	Tarlene Lotion
	Tegrin Lotion
COAL TAR GELS:	Aquatar
	Estar
	P&S Plus
	PsoriGel
COAL TAR FOR COMPOUNDING:	Rx Crude Coal Tar
	LCD (solution)
	Tar Distillate Doak (solution)
	Rx Zetar Emulsion
OTHER:	Boyol ointment
	Ichthammol ointment
	Tarpaste
	Rx 20-10-5 Lotion

*Coal tar strength expressed in terms of crude coal tar equivalency to allow a rough comparison of strength. Actual product may use coal tar solution, distillate, extract, etc., and these preparations differ somewhat in terms of their therapeutic properties.

Strength*	Size
0.1, 0.25 ,0.5%	50 gm
1%	50 gm
0.25, 0.5%	50 gm
0.1, 0.2, 0.4%	65 gm
1%	65 gm
0.1, 0.25, 0.5, 1%	45 gm
0.4%	60 gm
0.1, 0.2, 0.3, 0.4%	Compounded
1% (+1.7% Allantoin)	60 gm
2%	85,454 gm
0.18% (+1% SA, 1% resorcinol, 0.5% benzoic acid)	52.5,90 gm
1%	60,132 gm
1, 3, 5%	Compounded
1%	480 gm
0.4% (+1.5% sulfur, 1.5% SA)	120,480 gm
1%	480 gm
5% (+5% Ammoniated mercury, 2% methenamine sulfosalicylate)	60,480 gm
1% (+1.7% Allantoin)	240 ml
2.5%	240 ml
5.2%	120 ml
5%	120 ml
2% (+2% SA)	60 ml
1.5%	125 ml
9.7% (+2% Benzocaine, 1% SA)	57,120 ml
2%	60 ml
1%	180 ml
0.5%	90 gm
5%	90 gm
1.6% (+2% SA)	105 gm
1.5%	120 gm
100%	
20%	
20% (Distilled: nonstaining)	60,480 ml
30% (Crude coal tar)	180 ml
10% Ichthammol (+Benzocaine)	30 gm
10, 20%	30,480 gm
5% Coal tar in Lassar's paste	30,120 gm
20% Juniper tar (Oil of Cade)- (+10% Sulfur, 5% SA)	Compounded

FU = fluorouracil
LA = lactic acid
MA = monochloracetic acid

SA = salicylic acid
TA = trichloroacetic acid

Brand Name	Generic
Acu-Sol solution	2% glutaraldehyde
Rx Bichloracetic acid	Dichloroacetic acid
Rx Cantharone	0.7% cantharidin
Rx Cantharone Plus	30% SA, 5% podophyllin, 1% cantharidin
Cidex, Cidex 7 solution	2% glutaraldehyde
Rx Compound W solution	14% SA, 11% acetic acid
gel	
Rx Condylox solution	0.5% podofilox
Derma-soft cream	2.5% SA
Rx Duofilm solution	16.7% SA, 16.7% LA
Rx Duoplant gel	27% SA
Rx Efudex cream	5% 5-FU
solution	2.5% 5-FU
Rx Fluoroplex cream	1% 5-FU
solution	1% 5-FU
Formadon	10% formaldehyde
Rx Formaray	20% formaldehyde
Freezone solution	13.6% SA
Glutaraldehyde	2–20% glutaraldehyde
Rx Gordofilm	16.7% SA, 16.7 LA
Rx Lactisol solution	16.7% SA, 16.7 LA
Rx LazerFormalyde	10% formaldehyde
Mediplast	40% SA plaster
Rx Mono-Chlor	80% MA
Rx Occlusal solution	17% SA
Rx Occlusal HP solution	26% SA
Off-Ezy solution	17% SA
Rx Pod-Ben-25	25% podophyllin
Rx Salacid ointment	25% SA in petrolatum
	60% SA in petrolatum
Salactic film	16.7% SA, 16.7% LA
Rx TI-Flex solution	17% SA, 17% LA
Transplantar pads (20 mm)	22% SA (Karaya gum dermal delivery)
Rx Trans-versal pads (6 or 12 mm)	15% SA (Karaya gum dermal delivery)
Rx Tri-Chlor	50–80% TA
Rx Verr Canth	0.7% cantharidin
Rx Verrex	10% podophyllin, 30% SA
Rx Verrusol	5% podophyllin, 30% SA, 1% cantharidin
Rx Viranol solution	16.7% SA, 16.7% LA
gel	12% SA
Wart-Off solution	17% SA

Note: Tretinoin (Retin-A) has been used effectively on flat warts. (See: Acne Medications)

size	Dose
960,3840 ml	3×/wk
.5,75 ml	> or = qwk
7.5 ml	Up to 24h, up to 6h (molluscum)
7.5 ml	Up to 24h
960,3840 ml	3×/wk
10 ml	qd
7.5 gm	
3.5 ml	bid 3d/wk
30 gm	qd
15 ml	qd
14 gm	qd
25 mg	bid
10 ml	bid
30 gm	bid
30 ml	bid
45,120,1920,3840 ml	bid
45,120 ml	bid
9.3 ml	qd
480 ml (25%)	3×/wk
15 ml	qd
15 ml	qd
90 ml	bid
25/box	qd
15 ml	> or = qwk
15 ml	qd
10 ml	qd
13.3 ml	qd
30 ml	12h (1–6h genital)
60,480 gm	
60 gm	
15 ml	qd
15 ml	qd
25/box	qd
40/box	qd
15 ml	> or = qwk
7.5 ml	Up to 24h, up to 6h (molluscum)
7.5 ml	12h (1–6h genital)
7.5 ml	up to 24h
10 ml	qd
8 gm	qd
15 ml	qd

Acetic Acid	(1–5%) 5% acetic acid lowers bacterial count in infected wounds and is often used in infections involving *Pseudomonas aeruginosa*.
Bluboro tabs	Aluminum sulfate, calcium acetate (boxes of 12, 100 tabs)
Buro-Sol powder	Aluminum acetate (Burow's solution) (boxes of 12, powder 120 gm)
Domeboro powder (also: Bluboro, Pedi-Boro Soak Paks)	Aluminum sulfate, calcium acetate (Burow's solution) (boxes of 12, 100 pkts)
Domeboro tabs	Aluminum sulfate, calcium acetate (Burow's solution) (boxes of 12,100,1000 tabs)
Oxyzal	Oxyquinolone sulfate, benzalkonium Cl (1:2000) (30,120,480 ml)
Potassium permanganate	(0.025–0.1%). Causes stains.
Rx Silver nitrate	(0.1–0.5%). Causes stains. If used as wet dressing over extensive area, can cause hyponatremila or hypochloremia. 10, 20, 50% products and silver nitrate applicator sticks used to destroy exuberant granulation tissue or as caustic agents (10, 20, 50% solutions—30 ml each) (10% ointment—30 gm).

NOTE:

(1) *Domeboro* or *Bluboro:* 1 packet or 1 tablet per pint of water
   = 1:40 solution
   (2 packets/pint water = 1:20 solution)
   (4 packets/pint water = 1:10 solution)

(2) *Buro-Sol:* 1 packet per pint of water = 1:15 solution

(3) All of the preparations on this page are astringents and antibacterial agents. Potassium permanganate also is fungicidal.

1. Cardinale VA, ed. Drug topics red book (annual pharmicists reference). 93rd ed. Oradell, NJ: Medical Economics Co. Inc., 1989.

2. Huff BB, ed. Physician's desk reference. 43rd ed. Oradell, NJ: Medical Economics Co. Inc., 1989.

3. Huff BB, ed. Physician's desk reference for nonprescription drugs. 10th ed. Oradell, NJ: Medical Economics Co. Inc., 1988.

4. Olin BR, ed. Drug facts and comparisons. St. Louis: Facts and Comparisons, a division of the J.B. Lippencott Co., 1989.

5. Arndt KA. Manual of dermatologic therapeutics. 4th ed. Boston: Little, Brown and Company, 1987.

6. Gilman AG, Goodman LS, Gilman A, eds. The pharmacologic basis of therapeutics. 7th ed. New York: Macmillan Publishing Co., Inc., 1985.

7. Mullins JD. Medicated applications. In: Osol A, ed. Remington's pharmaceutical sciences. 16th ed. Easton, PA: Mack Publishing Company, 1980.

8. Sanford JP. Guide to antimicrobial therapy 1988. W. Bethesda, MD: Jay P. Sanford, M.D., 1988.

9. Gupta MA, Gupta AK, Haberman HF. Psychotropic drugs in dermatology. J Am Acad Dermatol 1986;14:633–645.

10. Baer RL. Papavarine therapy in atopic dermatitis. J Am Acad Dermatol 1985;13:806–808.

11. Meinking TL, Taplin D, Kalter D, Eberle MW. Comparative efficacy of treatment for pediculosis capitis infections. Arch Derm 1986;122:267–271.

12. Frosch PJ, Kligman AM. The soap chamber tests: a new method for assessing the irritancy of soaps. J Am Acad Dermatol 1979;1:35–41.

13. Roenigk HH Jr, Auerbach R, Maibach HI. Methotrexate in psoriasis: revised guidelines. J Am Acad Dermatol 1988;19:145–156.

14. Krusinski PA. Treatment of mucocutaneous herpes simplex infections with acyclovir. J Am Acad Dermatol 1988;18:179–181.

15. Conant MA. Prophylactic and suppressive treatment with acyclovir and the management of herpes in patients with acquired immunodeficiency syndrome. J Am Acad Dermatol 1988;18:186–188.

16. Arndt KA. Adverse reactions to acyclovir: topical, oral, and intravenous. J Am Acad Dermatol 1988;18:188–190.

17. Huff JC. Antiviral treatment in chickenpox and herpes zoster. J Am Acad Dermatol 1988;18:204–206.

18. Ellis CN, Vorhees JJ. Etretinate therapy. J Am Acad Dermatol 1987;16:267–291.

19. Strauss JS, Rapini RP, Shalita AR, et al. Isotretinoin therapy for acne: results of a multicenter dose-response study. J Am Acad Dermatol 1984;10:490–496.

20. Leyden JJ, James WD. *Staphylococcus aureus* infection as a complication of isotretinoin therapy. Arch Dermatol 1987;123:606–608.

21. Lebowitz MA, Berson DS. Ocular effects of oral retinoids. J Am Acad Dermatol 1988;19:209–211.

22. Kilcoyne RF. Effects of retinoids in bone. J Am Acad Dermatol 1988;19:212–216.

23. Strauss JS. Sebaceous Glands. In: Fitzpatrick TB, Eisen AZ, Wolff K, et al. eds. Dermatology in general medicine. 3rd ed. New York: McGraw-Hill, Inc., 1987.

24. Fisher AA. Contact Dermatitis. 3rd ed. Philadelphia: Lea and Febiger, 1986.

25. Smoot EC, Kucan JO. Management of soft tissue wound infections with topical antibacterials. Res Staff Physician 1987;33:27–33.

26. Berk MA, Lorincz AL. The treatment of bullous pemphigoid with tetracycline and niacinamide. Arch Dermatol 1986;122:670–674.

27. Smith BH, Bogoch S, Dreyfus J. The broad range of clinical use of phenytoin. New York: Dreyfus Medical Foundation, 1988.

28. Dandruff, seborrheic dermatitis, and psoriasis drug products for over-the-counter human use: tentative final monograph. Federal Register 1986;51:286–300.

29. Lesher JL, Smith JG Jr. Antifungal agents in dermatology. J Am Acad Dermatol 1987;17:383–394.

30. Bickers DR, Hagen PG, Lynch WS. Clinical pharmacology of skin diseases, New York: Churchill-Livingstone Press, 1984.

31. Picascia DD, Garden JM, Freinkel RK, Roenigk HH Jr. Treatment of resistant psoriasis with systemic cyclosporine. J Am Acad Dermatol 1987;17:408–414.

32. Ellis CN, Gorsulowsky DG, Hamilton TA, et al. Cyclosporine improves psoriasis in a double-blind study. JAMA 1986;256:3110–3116.

33. Biren CA, Barr RJ. Dermatologic applications of cyclosporine. Arch Dermatol 1986;122:1028–1032.

34. Sauermann G, Doerschner A, Hoppe U, Wittern P. Comparative study of skin care efficiency and in-use properties of soap and surfactant bars. J Soc Cosmet Chem 1986;37:309–327.

35. Tolman EL. Acne and Acneiform Dermatoses. In: Moschella SL, Hurley HJ, eds. Dermatology. 2nd ed. Philadelphia: W.B. Saunders Company, 1985.

Note: Items in *italics* are generic medications.